STANDING IN SPACE

Editor: Catherine Courtenaye
Photograph Restoration and Editing: Norrie Syme
Front Cover Photograph: Rachel Robertson, rachelrobertson.com
Interior Photographs: See credits within
Cover & Interior Design: Erin Burke

Production: Northern Summit Studio

Barry Lopez quotes taken from *Artic Dreams*:
pages 12, 321, 348 and 516. ISBN 0-684-18578-4.

For information on ordering, please visit **www.sixviewpoints.com**

Artcraft Printers, Billings, Montana
Printed in the United States of America

ISBN: 978-1-5136-1361-1

Fallon Press

FIRST PRINTING

5 4 3 2 1

Standing in Space

The Six Viewpoints Theory & Practice

Mary Overlie

to all artists deep in thought

&

to my brother Eric

Preface

Acknowledgments

Preface

THIS BOOK IS STYLED AS A SERIES OF SOCRATIC DIALOGUES interrogating the stage and performance as natural phenomena. Folded into these dialogues you will find: (a) a curriculum setting out a progression of study; (b) the relevant history in order to understand the intent of this study; and (c) a complete Practice Manual describing the Viewpoints classroom practices, each followed by descriptions of the desired results. Such a structure allows the Six Viewpoints to be integrated into a nonhierarchical pedagogical and artistic practice. Nonhierarchical refers to any situation characterized by impartiality.

The Viewpoints approach both dance and theater as physical entities akin to natural landscapes that can be entered and traversed. In this specific gaze at the art form of performance, creating plays or choreographies in the traditional sense is not directly addressed. These two creative entities are left in the hands of the artists with the hope that the Viewpoints shed some light on their individual practices. In other words, the Six Viewpoints do not offer up a safari through the landscape of performance as a relatable, convenient and safe journey for the traveler. The Viewpoints is dedicated to reading the stage as a force of nature. Culling the experiences of performance like a mountain climber, the performer explores the basic material with their own body, their own presence.

Always deeply reflective and independently minded as a child, I once thought I would be a painter like my beloved next door neighbors. I grew up physically embedded in nature and mentally enthralled with art. When I discovered dance, the two came together: I thought about choreography as painting with my body, and as I advanced I discovered that the stage was half canvas and half mountain. That the walls of the theater were like canyons, the visual presence of the body like shapes of boulders and trees, movement was the same as the kinetic world of the rivers and the wind. That time moved on and on from second to millennium, from the beginning of time to encircling me in my breathing, that emotion was present in my presence, and that logic or story was there before I entered the space. I set about looking for the languages to express this existence, the materials of my performance world. The phenomenological nature of this journey, now called the Six Viewpoints, allows me to question what is present in traditional forms and what lies beneath and beyond formal art.

> "The physical landscape is baffling in its ability to transcend whatever we would make of it. It is as subtle in its expression as turns of the mind, and larger than our grasp; and yet it is still knowable. The mind, full of curiosity and analysis, disassembles a landscape and then reassembles the pieces—the nod of a flower, the color of the night sky, the murmur of an animal—trying to fathom its geography. At the same time the mind is trying to find its place within the land, to discover a way to dispel its own sense of estrangement."
>
> BARRY LOPEZ, *Arctic Dreams*

The Six Viewpoints' regard for the stage as a physical entity allows us to encounter information before the creative act of making. By a specific process of deconstruction, six materials located as the Six Viewpoints—Space, Shape, Time, Emotion, Movement and Story—are separated from the creative act and emerge as conversations. This dialogue includes but does not favor the actor, dancer, choreographer or director over the materials of performance. In the process of discovering the languages of these materials, they are placed on an equal footing. As this occurs, just as in these quoted passages by Barry Lopez, an element of estrangement between the performer, the stage and the audience is dissolved.

"The beauty here is a beauty you feel in your flesh. You feel it physically.... Other beauty takes only the heart, or the mind."

"... this affinity for the land, I believe, is an antidote to the loneliness that in our own culture we associate with individual estrangement and despair."

BARRY LOPEZ, *Arctic Dreams*

The Six Viewpoints grew out of observations and experiments that have been organized into a systematic approach to performance. The drive to find this structure is part of my evolution as an artist and reflects the philosophical, social and spiritual influences of my childhood and of an era that made great strides creating new languages in many fields of art.

The work of Philip Glass in music; Richard Serra, Richard Nonas, Donald Judd in sculpture; Dan Flavin and Keith Sonnier in painting/visual arts; Yvonne Rainer, Barbara Dilley, Trisha Brown, Lucinda Childs, Steve Paxton and Stephen Petronio in dance; Robert Wilson, Richard Foreman, Joanne Akalitis, Liz LeCompte and Lee Breuer in theater are all extraordinary examples of an era of esthetic game-changing art. From my perspective these artists investigated their art forms through a natural, phenomenological interrogation of their mediums, deviating from the traditional path of creative invention. My favorite art of the 1970s focused awareness on the most basic materials, seeking art that could be found in what already existed in the forms before the artist is even present. This work was dedicated to bringing these fragile and profound sources to the audience.

The Viewpoints evolution draws on many sources:

- my childhood in Montana

- my teachers in a new age of dance

- the atmosphere of the SoHo art scene of the seventies where I lived and worked

- dance artists whose work, I believe, was interrogating their own bodies as physical/natural phenomenon

- my many years of choreographing and performing

- my many years of teaching: at the Internationale Tanzwochen Wien in Vienna, Austria; other locations in Europe and America; and as full-time faculty of the Experimental Theatre Wing, which I helped create at Tisch School of the Arts Undergraduate Drama, New York University

This book follows my esthetic of allowing students, artists and the audiences to find their own way. You will find no formulas or directions about how to make good theater or dance. In my opinion, art and the experience of viewing art must come with a challenge: to re-learn what is already known. If students are given a solid foundation in the process of interrogating, along with viable technical skills to meet the conditions of interrogation, they will be able to find new truths and new perspectives, and the audience will be able to follow their findings.

- The Viewpoints training:

- launches students on their own physical interrogation of the materials

- discusses results of investigations

- proposes challenges to make new discoveries

The Practice Manual at the conclusion of this book is designed to bring together artist, audience and the materials of performance.

The art of performance has been analyzed and theorized over many generations in the interest of improving and extending technical and artistic knowledge. The Six Viewpoints does not seek to challenge history or to replace it but to simply add to this knowledge. Directors, choreographers, actors and dancers have always worked with the materials that are being interrogated here. The title, Six Viewpoints, refers to a unique and radical emphasis on infinitesimally small particles of awareness.

Deconstruction of ever-narrowing iterations is used to separate the physical stage and physical performance into Space, Shape, Time, Emotion, Movement and Story. Separating the form exposes a different plane of knowledge, one that allows for a new integration of the materials.

The interrogation of art can be broken down into three distinct movements:

- the Classicists assumed that the stage was there to practice and celebrate form

- the Modernists assumed that the stage was there to examine the lives and difficulties of human existence

- the Postmodernists assume that the stage is there to enact microscopic interrogation of our physical, mental and emotional world

As a postmodern structure, the Viewpoints believe that:

- there is no need to add an extra narrative into performance, because performance is a dialogue with the natural elements themselves

- viewers have the visual and mental capacity to organize and understand what they are witnessing since they are familiar with the raw materials from the artists' daily life

- there is a message and intelligence before the artist arrives onstage

The Six Viewpoints contains a second structure, the Bridge, to accompany the natural investigation of materials (Space, Shape, Time, Emotions, Movement and Story, or SSTEMS). The Bridge is formulated from nine interrogations I conducted. It functions as a stimulus to investigation, as a way of substantiating the ideas surrounding the Viewpoints, and also contains a vital teaching curriculum. Each interrogation forms a laboratory aimed at understanding the practice of nonhierarchical treatment of the stage and performance. This series of laboratories create a type of double helix in which the six raw physical materials, the SSTEMS, are accompanied by conceptual guides that clarify the interrogations.

The traditional hierarchies of story/emotion in acting and movement/music in dancing are structures dictating the use and value of the rest of the stage's materials. The Six Viewpoints employs this double helix-like structure to require the artist to function as a trained observer, equal partner and free agent in conversation with all materials. A transition is required to discard the traditional creator/originator definition of the artist. The study of the SSTEMS and the Bridge is that transition.

The evolution of the Six Viewpoints came about as naturally as the study that they represent. Before I knew dance, I was a wild and unfettered child surrounded by the vast, "empty" spaces of Montana. I lived on a hillside that ran into mountains continuing for nearly a hundred miles straight into Yellowstone National Park. Anything in that landscape that could provide a chance to experience movement was irresistible: the hills to run on, the creek to float, the railroad track to balance on, the trees to hide between, grass to slide down on improvised cardboard sleds at breakneck speed, and sleds on snow in winter. Later would come skiing, mountain climbing and camping at high altitudes.

While still a child in Montana I developed a hunger to learn the technical languages of choreography. Impressed by discussions between fine art painters who lived across the road I embarked on my pursuit of a physical equivalent of ancient visual languages of perspective, entry of light on the canvas, dialogue between the center of canvas in relationship to the edges, etc. At 17 I ran away from home catching a freight train to San Francisco and at 24 was invited to join the New York City dance company Natural History of the American Dancer, Performing Lesser Known Species Volumes 12 thru 24 at the Whitney Museum of American Art. I moved to New York and carried out my search in three primary laboratories:

- the early SoHo galleries and artists' lofts where I witnessed and was involved in much creative outpouring

- intense improvisational rehearsal and performance with The Natural History of the American Dancer

- my own studio at 530 Canal Street, where I choreographed and improvised with my dance company

Each step of my journey is reflected in this interrogation of the SSTEMS and the Bridge.

PART ONE

MATERIALS:
THE SSTEMS

The SSTEMS

Space—Shape—Time—Emotions—Movement—Story

MATERIALS. THE VERY WORD MAKES ME WANT TO STRETCH MY JOINTS, engage my body and go to work. The project of the following six chapters is to bring a perspective to the materials of the stage and of performance, allowing these elements to take the lead in a creative dialogue. This action of affirmation emanating from the stage allows the artist/performer to reach beyond creative imagination. The Six Viewpoints invites a one-on-one, knowledgeable, integrated, physical relationship with the art of performance.

To begin, you might try the following curriculum: read each chapter on the SSTEMS and at the same time take each of the SSTEMS one at a time using each of the practices found in succession in the Practice Manual. In your approach follow this advice:

Turn off the impulse to control or own the material. Listen and see what already exists, instead of trying to manipulate a material into something that looks like art or theater or dance to you. Simply be there in it, be aware and be curious. This may be uncomfortable at first. It may also be a great relief. Getting to know the SSTEMS can impart a sense of freedom and connectedness based on a simple existence with what surrounds us.

Work very specifically with the individual material. Resist the impulse to add several SSTEMS to any practice unless you make a conscious choice to mix focuses. This is critical to hone your awareness and understanding of each separate material.

Gather as much "useless" data as you can. This information may in fact seem contrary to the desire to make art. It is with this useless data that your can tune in the languages of the SSTEMS.

Take time to explore. This interrogation requires time to allow the body to absorb information. The length of time it takes to become a good SSTEMS linguist will vary from person to person, but I recommend at least 36 hours of data collection in each SSTEMS as a good starting point. Your learning will accumulate naturally without an objective and you will be in conversations that can lead you somewhere.

CHAPTER 1

Space

Cleared of the clutter of plays and choreographies, what remains onstage? What lies beneath inventions? To locate the first of the materials, Space, try to find a nonhierarchical perspective by warming up your body so it is fully awake, then climb into Space by simply standing, walking, observing, listening and feeling the space you have at hand. Entering into a physical relationship to Space takes time and you should use every means available to explore and familiarize yourself with this material. Run your hands over the walls and floor, turn at every angle by increments of an inch and see what you are facing. Measure the Space you have entered using the tools of mathematics as my father used to map roads, lay out crops and later hunt for oil. Use your body to begin to know the distances in the room by how many aikido rolls it takes to cross from end to end; walk all the steps in every diagonal.

As you do these practices a catalogue of awarenesses will form and become a part of your physical and visual life as a performer. Find the center. Relocate the center and experiment with what happens to the rest of the Space when you do so. As you engage in this manner you will begin to merge with the Space and be allowed to receive its "thinking," its "art," its "voice." As you begin to measure, Space will take on the ability to direct you, and your visual perceptions will begin to scan a much more profound level of spatial awareness.

With these explorations, the Six Viewpoints is passing on investigations that are the direct result of my own introduction to Space in 1970, in the midst of the Conceptual Minimalist art movement. Walk through a perceptual door to Space, and it begins to be your partner in performance. Standing in Space onstage removes a kind of alienation that can sometimes cause a feeling of loneliness and insecurity. As you become aware that you have a profound material as a collaborator these feelings depart and an integration with Space becomes something that is with you at all times onstage.

With an invitation to come to New York to participate in an exciting new kind of dance based in improvisation, a vivid and life-changing realization was hovering just around a conceptual corner from me. The work being done at that time in music, sculpture, painting, theater and dance still resonates throughout the art world with its radically stripped down nature of the experimentation.

You could say Space was in my blood, coming from Montana, but what began to draw an awareness of Space as a dancer was a solo given to me by Barbara Dilley. She was giving a workshop in San Francisco, having left the Merce Cummingham Dance Company just a few years earlier and currently performing with the ensemble The Grand Union. I had no thoughts of going to New York, enraptured as I was with mountain climbing in the Sierras and dancing in the open air by the Bay. Although I must admit, I was terribly lonely as an artist and bored, lacking artistic stimulus. Dilley's solo was, I believe, her first choreography, created for herself in 1968 and titled Blind Bird Box Dance. It was based on the concept of "dancing the energies in the space." And those were my instructions.

I was to rehearse on my own in a beautiful studio full of light. I went through weeks of hell not knowing what I was looking for and where to start. I would leave the studio feeling dizzy and nauseated by the presence of so much space and nothing to do in it. I resolved the problem by studying aikido. I cannot remember whether Barbara had suggested this or not. Aikido directs the energy of the space and of the opponent's movements as a combated skill. I began to be able to perceive the energy flow in my rehearsal studio and eventually could work for hours just letting it push my body as a part of the flow. I had gained an invisible dance partner/choreographer.

Barbara seemed pleased with my performance and I was rewarded with an invitation to come to New York to work with her on her next project, a performance at the Whitney Museum. For my part I was impressed with how a simple thing like Space could be so engaging to perform. Much to my amazement, I had located Space and had begun to grapple with this material. I had not discovered that it was possible to encounter it as a discrete focus beyond a specific dance.

Any student of the Six Viewpoints, once they have begun to discover Space through "standing in it," must immediately begin to test its efficacy as a performance medium. Just as the artists in SoHo in the seventies, myself included, discovered, you must establish that a performance based on Space will work. You need to test Space to see how it responds as an effective communicative language. For this you need the Petri dish of a community where you can make small works and perform them for an audience. Through direct testing you find your guides. Like taking a boat through the Northwest Passage, you have to be in a situation where you are called upon to make your communication with Space work. You need to test if your skill with Space passes as art or not. I tell my students, "Let the materials teach you. They know more and have better ideas." Certainly the Space of so many stages has taught me and continues to teach me to work with the thrill of its physical presence.

All performance techniques—and Space is a performance technique, just as there are mountaineering techniques, ice flow navigation techniques, and ballet—must be tested for efficacy by the artists who use them. No progress can be made by copying a look or a formula when it comes to making your own work with the raw materials.

Although I had studied Cunningham technique and felt a part of his influence, I finally met Merce Cunningham as a participant in one of the Pro Series in the late 1980s. He and his company were performing their entire repertory as the basis of the Vienna Summer Dance Festival, the Tanzwochen Wien. Some years later in the early 1990s he came to teach a workshop for the Pro Series at the Tanz Wochen, a project for which I was partially responsible for setting up.

At this workshop he introduced his 360-degree use of Space. This concept had evolved, out of his collaborations with filmmaker Charles Atlas, to address his frustrations in having to alter his choreography to suit the confined space of a camera lens.

As a part of the Pro Series Workshops, I led a kind of study group that worked on coming up with insightful questions for interviewing choreographers visiting the festival. The evening of our arranged talk with Merce Cunningham, one of my students asked him if he ever got tired of what he was doing. He said yes. There was a gasp from the audience at the audacity of the question and also at his reply. Then he very earnestly told us that when that happened, he took a walk around the block and he was back to work. I believe that he was in his late seventies at the time. That kind of dedication is only found when the artist has tested their work and found it to be valuable. If their interrogation of the materials and concept they have chosen is well founded, the dialogue is inexhaustible.

Looking back I can see how the process of comprehending this material was slowly wearing away my inherited dance self-involvement. I was beginning to shed bad habits that had materialized as space blockers: dance techniques and choreographies that filled the Space with movements lacking any deep relationship to the studio or the stage. At the time I moved to New York, after Blind Bird Box Dance, I would not have been able to issue the instructions at the opening of this chapter. I still had no comprehension of the cascade of deconstructing, "particalizing," nonhierarchical epiphanies that were to follow. Almost four months after I moved to New York, in a rehearsal at 112 Green Street with the Natural History of the American Dancer company, I found myself joining Suzie Harris singing "au naturel, au naturel, we want to be au naturel!" We were celebrating our efficiency as readers of the natural elements in the stage. For me that process had begun in earnest with our rehearsals for the Whitney concert.

We rehearsed virtually every day in a completely nonverbal artistic meeting. Like mountain climbing, you begin and work your way through. The spoken word has nothing to do with it. Space emerged as a clear language of our dancing. We were given the time to discover it with our bodies as it emerged on its own. Space came with its own languages, such as heightened awareness of visual patterns and connections. All of the SSTEMS slowly emerged with their own nonverbal languages and principles appearing out of the physical engagement with the dancing. The dancers were

Barbara Dilley, Rachael Lew, Suzie Harris, Cynthia Hedstrom, Carmen Beauchat, Judy Padow and myself. We came into the studio and researched with no formal instructions or imaginings of what we were looking for. To me this is the ultimate artistic freedom. And we found so much from willingness, thoughtfulness and diligence.

As has happened often over the years, after our first public performances that year at the Whitney, I was proud of the enlightenment I had achieved. Unknown to me at the time, as a dancer I was far from a true understanding of Space. I had acquired an intense relationship and love of Space and had begun to comprehend that I had entered into a sort of village within an art movement. I was finding out the languages and secret methods of its practices. The inhabitants of this village, my fellow dancers and artists of every medium, would attend each other's performances, ad hoc painting and sculpture openings, and listen to new music compositions several nights a week. I remember hearing Philip Glass introduce his work as I sat on a folding chair in a parking lot, with the notes repeating and slowly rising to the sky in a spiral it seemed. At the same time, my project, what would come to be known as the Six Viewpoints, was collecting more and more deconstructive structural information. The materials emerging in our rehearsals would be labeled the six SSTEMS. The SSTEMS, the six viewpoints through which to enter performance, would form the name of this philosophy and practice.

We had had a wonderful and intense time at the Whitney Museum. Communicating in that way with that group of women was a deeply formative experience for all of us. When the performance was over we wanted to extend our work, and formed a collective performance group under Barbara's original title, The Natural History of the American Dancer. We decided that each of us would make and perform a solo to officially introduce ourselves to each other. The beauty of Space had been weaving in and out of our work for months so I decided to make a solo in an unusual place to show my admiration for the material. I would soon learn just how much less educated and newer to the scene I was than the other six women.

Still fresh from California, I thought it would be smart and "avant-garde" if I did a solo outdoors. So there I was, standing across the street from the gallery at 112

Greene Street, where we most often rehearsed on the second floor, Suzie Harris's loft . When I finished my dance there was a terrible silence from the company. The thought passed through my mind that I had just finished my association with them. I was out! Then Suzy asked Rachael if she wanted to make a comment. No, Rachael did not want to speak. So Suzy asked me: "Do you know where you are?"

I was shocked. What a question. I said that I was in New York City. She said, "Yes, but do you know where you are?" I began to panic. I could not imagine what she meant. Finally Rachael said, "You are about two feet from the building behind you, three-quarters up the block, and 12 feet from the building across the street." In that instant I was transported from a partial, performance use of Space to a much greater understanding of Space. I realized that I could have a dialogue with Space as a discrete material. The final act of deconstruction fell into place and I came to occupy a position as an artist in this vast material. SHAZZAM!!!

A few days later I returned to Montana to spend the summer studying "where I was." I had entered into a lifelong dialogue with this exquisite material. My research began in the unrelenting horizons of treeless prairie 30 miles from the Canadian border. I remember standing in my parents' kitchen in Shelby, Montana: The table is up against the wall below the window. I am at a very odd angle to the room . . . . After a month, I began to truly see and feel Space. Once back in New York with our company, I extended my research in rehearsals and in performance. Later I would choreograph with Space and teach others about "Space consciousness." I had found the first of six materials that are the foundation of Viewpoints theory.

As you explore Space outside of its use in theater or dance, a profound realization, a performance presence, settles into your being. That presence is the consciousness of standing in Space on a visual and interactive plane that overlaps the performing and visual arts. With practice, you gain the means to tip your work in any direction by placing more or less emphasis on Space. A choreography can be based primarily on spatial patterns, as in the work of Lucinda Childs and her complicated counting. Her ensemble, using only steps and skipping, with arms held low in an almost pedestrian manner to reduce their visual impact, performed Space as a visual/dimensional entity. Her work with Space broke barriers in dance, and the art form crossed over into visual arts territory. The same dramatic effect can be witnessed in the works of Robert Wilson. His use of Space as one of the main sources of narrative has given his work worldwide and operatic impact. He is respected in both performance and the visual arts as a groundbreaking artist.

As a performer, there is nothing quite like being trained to consciously stand in Space without depending on elaborate movement, music, story or character. Both Childs and Wilson require dancers able to perform this task. Historically, Space was subordinated to the story and used as blocking, or arranged primarily to fill the needs of the onstage movement. When a one-on-one relationship with Space is fully realized, Space awareness itself can become a primary artistic driver of the performance. The fully developed relationship with Space is not a "skill" that can be simply copied stylistically. Hours of standing in Space is required to truly occupy the stillness, to hold the action of Space.

As you read through this chapter and encounter any difficulty in understanding Space as a discrete material, remember that there is nothing fundamentally unfamiliar in the concept. Understanding Space is an innate ability that most of us possess to varying degrees. Investigating Space through the Six Viewpoints, along with the other materials in the SSTEMS, is direct and obvious. When you add observation of distances between yourself and fellow performers, and pay attention to the spatial patterns you make together, you will develop an awareness of Space as a unifying effect. The practice of Space awareness has been in use since the seventies to instill ensemble performance skills.

In contrast to marching in drill formation or other externally directed ways of forming an ensemble, the Viewpoints' acute spatial awareness introduces a practice that functions as a self-directed language. A dialogue free of external instructions brings performers into a unique dynamic unity. Focusing on such basic elements as "where am I, where is everyone else, where are the walls, where are we going, what does this look like spatially to the audience?" can achieve a particular unity while maintaining individual independent perspective. "Listening" to Space starts with a conversation that gathers into a heightened sense of cooperation.

When you are teaching the Viewpoints or rehearsing with performers who do not know the Viewpoints, it is easy to see which performers are not familiar with or are having difficulty with becoming aware of Space. Without a developed spatial perception, they unconsciously behave as if they are the center of attention. Performers who lack spatial awareness tend to gravitate towards the center of the stage, are not able to perceive the placement of others as important information and do not experience any visual impact of their own movements in Space. Space is only where they are and center stage just seems the right place to stand, since the rest of the stage feels empty and meaningless. Rooted in one spot, these performers are immobilized and deliver their lines or dance moves with one spatial focus. They have a tendency to fixate on their scene or dance partners rather than on the pattern between them. In their minds, a partner is the only other important focus since they are surrounded by useless voids. It is always amazing to me that to recover from this space blindness, all that is needed is a session or two of "Walk and Stop in Space" with the suggestion to observe and interact with what is surrounding them. For most of my students it is simply a case of waking up something they once knew intrinsically.

In traditional theater, a traditionally spatially aware actor might have a dialogue like this:

> "I am standing upstage left; I want to cross downstage right to sit in a chair. When I proceed in the opposite direction first, just a few steps, it enlivens the space and emphasizes the crossing toward the audience. The arc temporarily takes me closer to the other performer, gives me more time to say my line and gives me a variety of angles to make eye contact from. I can also look back at the space I just left, signifying a slight feeling of regret."

He or she is still using Space as blocking, although aware of the grace it affords their needs. If, however, the performer can trust in the articulation of Space as a full material, the "cross" to the chair could become something like this:

> "Wanting to sit in a chair but turning the hierarchy of the Space into a horizontal experience, I arrange to have the chair moved to three locations and I finally sit

down. Now I have the other characters arrange all the furniture to be in exactly the same relationship to the new position so that everything is now in the original position but the entire set has been adjusted to a new orientation onstage. Space is now alive as an important part of the piece of theater and the audience is alerted to the possibility that anything might happen."

Some years ago, a group of my students were working with Space in a small park in New York City, opposite the city's great spatial landmark, the Flatiron Building. It was lunchtime on a beautiful day. My students were practicing being invisible, so as not to impact or disturb the dining office workers crowded on the pathways and benches. The work was going quite well, and no one seemed to notice the students walking in strange patterns, stopping in various formations, sitting, and lying down to change their vertical relationship to street lamps, water fountains, and statues. This went on for 15, 20 minutes, with everything flowing smoothly. Then a woman pushing a baby carriage came to an abrupt stop a few feet away, transfixed, with an intense, concentrated energy on her face. Not only could she see all of the students within the crowd, but she seemed to fully and intuitively comprehend what they were doing!

I was curious about what caused the cloak of invisibility to drop so easily as she approached. I explained that we were a theater class from NYU. The woman turned with a bewildered, almost beatific glint in her eyes and said, "Since my baby was born I haven't had any space. For months and months, just me and the child. You and your students have given back to me a sense of space. Thank you. Thank you." As she walked off, pushing the stroller at a calm, leisurely pace, her body seemed to open up to the world around her. At that moment I felt a flash of profound gratitude to Space and what I had come to know about it. How elegant and communal it can be. How essential to life it is, how playful and important for our minds and for a healthy presence on the planet. While we were trying to keep to ourselves inconspicuous working in Space, she saw us the way a hungry person can smell food when others who are well fed cannot. She was able to see Space because she was in great need of it.

CHAPTER 2

Shape

THE VIEWPOINTS BEGIN TO LOCATE THE MATERIAL OF SHAPE THROUGH
detailed scrutiny of the physical/visual aspect of your own body. The interrogation
is established through a simple observation of symmetry, asymmetry, curvilinear
or angular forms. The observation of comparative placement of limbs, torso,
head, feet, hands, etc., reveals a link between the performer to all man-made and
natural structures. Breaking with traditional formal Shape training imparted to
performers mainly through dance techniques, martial arts and to some extent
Grotowski's Plastiques, Viewpoints Shape training creates a performative self-
awareness free of repetition. Seemingly awkward, at first this physical examination/
contemplation draws the performer past existing creative manipulations of Shape
into the infinite realm of Shape's own imagination, releasing self-consciousness,
egoism and narcissism.

Shape observation begins with a minimalistic "particalized" level of awareness.
Evolving out of our rehearsals for that first Natural History of the American
Dancer concert at the Whitney Museum, the language of Shape began to emerge
as one of the primary materials of performance and an important cornerstone in
the technical information I was seeking. As we rehearsed, if one of us assumed a
Shape, it would resonate in the other performer's Shape awareness, eventually
establishing a foundation for a physical structure of communication and design.

As any sculptor, potter, interior decorator or graphic designer will readily affirm, Shapes love to play with other Shapes. A vertical line will decide it likes another vertical line and then a twisted spiral resonates with the two and off we would go all the way into the most recent science of fractals. It is thrilling to participate in this primal dialogue.

As this dialogue evolves over time, the awareness of Shape transforms the performer, director or choreographer into an observer/participant in its languages. As this process takes place a performer often develops an unshakable confidence onstage no longer restricted by imagination, scripted or choreographed motivations and affirmed by the raw experienced Shape awareness. This transformation is brought about as performers realize that the very shape of their bodies is a medium of performance and is essentially art itself.

This realization for dancers can also inform more performative appreciation of the Shapes they are given in a choreography. For actors, the gestures—a much used aspect of Shape in acting—can take on greater variation and attention, becoming a significant part of performance rather than filler for the emotional or textual aspect of a play. Under this interrogation of the Shape of the physical self, a vast performative vocabulary, hiding in simple actions such as an arabesque, reaching for a glass of water, standing, or raising the arms, becomes recognizable and an important component of performative art.

In American theater, it is the work of playwright and director Richard Foreman that to me stands above all others as the most deeply evolved in the material of Shape. In his work, the carefully sculpted postures of the actors' bodies are what articulate their characters and also become their emotional subscripts. In his productions the objects, sets, costumes, and actors are all in one connective dialogue. Foreman's focus on Shape elevates props, set and costumes to equality with the actors. In his production Rhoda in Potato Land, 1975, the brilliant actress Kate Manheim was given oddly minimalist shapes that caused her to move with almost the same mobility as a potato. This lowly shape seemed to control everything that transpired, including emotions and narrative, in the awkward world she inhabited with stunning physical skill.

In the Natural History of the American Dancer, we found that Shape was a source for a type of abstract story/logic. A part of this discovery was a realization that Shape stories, approached through minimalistic physical scrutiny, did not confine us to a monotone agreement, as in the follow-the-leader practices sometimes found in other styles of improvisational training. Free as individuals, fully Shape-aware and connected like any two physical objects, performers can actively participate in Shape narrative, making the performance richer and vaster than passive copying could achieve. The physical and visual impact of repetition of form, if it should arise, is achieved from within the material itself rather than repeated as a practiced preordained form. Many years ago while thinking about these lessons I was struck by the similarity of this use of Shape to the invention of the corps de ballet by Russian choreographer Michel Folkine. We had been "inventing the wheel backwards" in the seventies, discovering connections that were made long ago in classic dance but with a twist of individual freedom.

This reading of Shape logic is something we naturally practice when hiking in the mountains or sailing on the ocean. We notice the patterns of the waves, the peaks, the snowflakes as a way of taking readings to know what is happening or what has happened long ago. Shape is a natural element in all sciences from geography to physics. Interrogating this material through a particle level of awareness, that is to say outside a preordained learned vocabulary, the performer is in a dialogue with Shape as an expansive form of communication.

A sense of calm and contemplation must be developed to apprehend this material. Objects, whether our bodies, a table, chair or bowl can only be deeply appreciated through a focus that has a meditative type of attention. Some years after I had become aware of Shape, the Origami Dance evolved: the folding and unfolding of the body, like a piece of paper, using my senses to appreciate the outcome, in what is like an endless flow of geometric possibilities suggested from one Shape becoming another, very much like the traditional practice of origami. Start with a simple fold in a piece of paper, or in this case the folding of a joint. Then with great patience study the fold and the Shape it has produced until you perceive the next. Shape creating Shape. This practice invokes what to me is one of the most fascinating parts of being an artist: the aspect of surrender.

In order to comprehend the power that Shape contains, I think it is valuable to consider the work of sculptor Richard Serra. My exposure to his work, beginning in the early gallery scene in SoHo, influenced my comprehension of the languages of Shape. At the time, the Natural History of the American Dancer was fully engrossed in working with the languages of Shape in our performances, and one evening, at a Serra opening, I felt an instant connection to his work. His regard for Shape seemed to match or run concurrent to our own amplifying role of the material.

The radical, bold simplicity of Serra's work was unlike anything I had ever experienced. I saw that his work engaged the Space through Shape and needed no other reason to exist. The massive forms sweep the viewer into participatory dialogue with Shape and Space. Unlike traditional sculpture, in Serra's work Shape stands not as a discrete object, but instead is felt through physical presence. You feel Shape and feel how it dictates the way you encounter Space. His work is a valuable lesson for the performer.

The impact of this exposure came out a few years later in my first full evening work, Painters Dream. The dance was sponsored by the Kitchen Center for Music and Dance, then housed on Grand Street in SoHo. The room was loft-like and elegant with four white columns and floor-to-ceiling arched windows overlooking the street. I decided to construct an abstract narrative made of a study of the Space itself, like a painter might study a canvas of a particular size and dimensions. The Shapes took form from the dimensions of the room itself.

I want to encourage dancers and choreographers to spend time with these materials in a totally nonhierarchical interrogation. When seen as an exclusive material, it appears to me that even dancers, who have tremendous training in Shape through various traditional techniques, tend to use a very limited Shape vocabulary compared to the plethora of shapes that are possible. When Shape's languages are confronted and explored, endless possibilities are opened.

The Six Viewpoints Shape awareness is an activity one usually associates with visual artists. Their studios are filled with objects that fascinate them. Their daily warm-up includes the perusal of these objects, their eye growing wise and more acute with each revisiting. They are not under the restraints and conditions of the temporal world of performance where we are under the impression that things must get done (and fast!). A visual artist will keep an object for years. And so, in the Viewpoints approach to this material, you can return to the practice of Shape awareness of your own body for years with ever increasing facility and awareness. Gennie DeWeese, my childhood art mentor, drew and painted the shapes from the same landscape outside her window on countless canvases, re-articulated the shapes of the Montana landscape in a non-ending, ever evolving discovery.

Now reach your hands out; look at them. Here is a Shape that is yours alone. Here is a material of performance existing in the form of your body. This material is both singular and universal. Begin by contemplating your own form. Simply take time—lots of time—to just look at your arms, your legs, and the position they are in, and their relationship to each other, as a painter would. Observe and wait for the moment when Shape begins to speak in Shape to you.

CHAPTER 3

Time

IN THE LATE SIXTIES AND EARLY SEVENTIES TIME BECAME A MAJOR element of an artistic and social revolution. Out the window went traditional performance/entertainment time and in came experiments with duration, repetition, non-accentuated beats and pedestrian-paced performance in music, dance, theater, sculpture, and the visual arts.

When I moved to SoHo I found myself at the core of a new use of Time both as a performer and as a spectator. I was astonished that I felt I had come home. It was as though the silence and rhythms of nature and emptiness of Montana had been transferred to SoHo. One of my favorite childhood occupations was watching, over many years, a pile of discarded two-by-fours slowly melt back into the earth. This fierce new art world was conducting Time experiments based in stillness and emptiness. Richard Nonas's sculptures had a deep connection to duration using his archaeological background and the ancient wood he worked with; the non-accented beats of text delivery by the Wooster Group's Ron Vawter; the pedestrian-paced dance of the Grand Union influenced by Yvonne Rainer; the endless repetition of musical chords by Philip Glass and Terry Riley; endless repetition of physical movements by Lucinda Childs and Dana Ritz; the dictates of time derived from the pendulum action of swinging motions as discovered by Trisha Brown and continued by Stephen Petronio; the nonlinear and unexcitable plays of Richard Foreman and Robert Wilson, and in his own way, Lee Breuer of Mabou Mines; and Judy Padow's choreographies based in walking patterns. All these experiments thereby delineating another approach to Time. You might call this approach Natural Cognitive Time. Or, as Barbara Dilley calls it, "The Elegant Pedestrian."

These experiments appeared to me to be artistic responses, set in motion by a slightly earlier call to the "tune in, turn on, and drop out" philosophy of the acid generation of Ken Kesey. As this artistic movement liberated itself from European conventions, Time found its own ground in an almost childlike simplicity and drifted toward Eastern contemplative philosophy. Although these experimental works appeared simple in form compared to traditional music and dance, they nonetheless evolved through, and require, arduous training and practice. A vital component of this experimentation was the retraining of the dancer, actor and musician to develop and maintain their own perception of Time without relying on the underlying beat (which traditionally would have been the narrative and lines of a play) or the dictates of a kinesthetic time signature through music. For me, this training began as a meditation. I added the practice of accepting walking (the organic pedestrian pace) as dancing. Paying a great deal of attention to walking, as though it were a long string of anatomical operations, allowed me to begin to inhabit Time as a free and exclusive material, separate from the other SSTEMS.

In many ways it can be argued that this specific interrogation of Time was one of the primary, embodied cores of the radical shifts taking place in the art movement of that era. In my lectures on the structure of the Six Viewpoints I express this shift, this emphasis on a contemplative Time, a natural Time, with a symbolic gesture: hand held out, palm cupped to receive while saying, "You see this, this is the Viewpoints, at any given time art will arrive on its own if you train yourself in observation and patience." This view of the practice of art embodies both a more conceptual and a more physical approach to Time. In order to bring about a perception of this type of Time, I retooled the practice of Walk and Stop (normally employed as an introduction to Space). Walk and Stop as a Time practice concentrates awareness on the length of time the practitioner stands, the length of time others stand and the length of time used to move from one place to another. I feel that, as the class practices Walk and Stop in Time, the whole classroom shifts location and we are in Montana with Time lapping at our feet as we walk up into the mountains and look across the plains.

In the patient lingering required in this version of Walk and Stop, you do not want to allow learned temporal habits to force a change of position. Hidden in this practice lurks an all-out attack on the overbearing rhythms that dominate music, traditional dance and drama, and socialized conversation. There is simply a time for standing and a time for walking. The objective of Walk and Stop in Time is to pull up and discard these roots of habitual social and artistic agreement. As you work in this practice, Time becomes a living, breathing, ephemeral material that unfolds itself so that you can physically inhabit it.

Although I worked with Time in its "natural" form, as duration, through six years of improvisation and five years of choreography, I began to realize, much to my annoyance, I still had not grasped the nature of this material. Although I knew the ecstasy of dancing without music, and then later experimented with using a magnificent classical score by making my choreography lay beside it in independent time signatures, I knew that Time itself seemed to be only defined by an outward activity. The questions kept hovering around me; there seemed to me a more basic level of Time that was eluding me. What was the inner connection, past activities, that thing that lies waiting for you on the stage even before you enter? This interrogation plagued me for years. I kept seeing a ghost tap dancer at the edge of my consciousness taunting me, hands on hips, staring at me, tap tap, tap . . . .

I knew that the question was still: how to go about apprehending Time? This idea of Time in the Viewpoints approach actually means entering into Time and developing a dialogue that can unlock all that might lend itself to performance. I found that I was still grappling with the most difficult road block, the calibration of Time in representational codes that break it into seconds, minutes, hours, dates, watches, calendars, metronomes, music scores. My recognition of duration had not been sufficient to remove the barrier that these systems created between me and Time.

The momentous occasion in which Time appeared to me came in October 1988, in Denmark, in the driveway of a house that was just outside the small village of calendars, metronomes, music scores. My recognition of duration had not been sufficient to remove the barrier that these systems created between me and Time.

The momentous occasion in which Time appeared to me came in October 1988, in Denmark, in the driveway of a house that was just outside the small village of Espergærde. I was taking the trash out. It was the day after I had gotten married. After planning a wedding while on tour the entire year, I was taking on a new partner, a new life and a new country. I thought I was fine. The wedding had been so much fun and so beautiful, people seemed happy.

Suddenly I found myself standing at the edge of the yard, trash strewn over the lawn. My clothes were dirty. I was totally lucid and calm, but then realized that I was a bit confused. There seemed to be a blank in my Time continuum. "Open the door, garbage in hand. Now standing, garbage all over the lawn?" I realized that "I" had been missing for some time. As I shook my head I began to realize that I had been on the ground, contorted in strange positions, catapulting through unplanned Space. I found that I was unhurt. It seems that I had been a puppy at play—they never get hurt as they jump and roll on their backs and slide and fall and fall and slide. Cool! Fast! I was moving so fast, so loose, so sure, that I did not think. I just was.

This phenomenon occurred several times over a period of two weeks, and I began to understand that I was experiencing fits of hysteria. In my hysterical fits, I was moving directly from my nervous system, without the filter of intentional, mental predetermination. Time was ripping through me, vibrating, a living entity, performing in the now! I discovered a kind of speed that fascinated me and I was suddenly aware that the measured and controlled time I normally lived in was a broken body-mind connection. I had exited a sluggish and indeterminate state of Time and had entered into an animal-like, immediate, accurate and vital Time that reached to my very core.

I spent the next two years working with hysteria-based speed in dance after dance. I learned how to train dancers to move into Time via their nervous system by extrapolating a practice from Bonnie Cohen's Body-Mind Centering (BMC) work: we develop our brain through movement patterns in a sequence that progresses from lower brain to midbrain to upper cortex. I have the students lie on the floor with back to the ground and suggest they attempt to move before thinking. This will result in rapid uncontrolled jerking of the body as the lower brain functions connect directly with the central nervous system to produce movement that is unfiltered by the higher cognitive functions of the mid- and forebrain. It is like jumpstarting a car—you are rerouting the habitual pathways or circuitry systems of the brain synapses. As the connection is made a rapid release of movements come coursing through the body, causing spurts of jerking, throwing and jumping that are both surprising and deeply satisfying, like touching something that has not been touched and wants to be used. I came to call this practice Automatic Movement. In it, you pass through borders of conventional acting and dancing Time and arrive at your own relationship to Time. As Automatic Movement is practiced it results in narrowing the synapses between body and mind, integrating the actor and dancer with Time. When you resume standing, your breathing is different. It is as though you are breathing directly into your nervous system instead of controlling the breath to fit a measured rhythm.

This Automatic Movement practice clears the pathway of body-mind communication and brings on a totally new way of feeling Time connected to the body. This "weird" experiment reveals Time in what I think of as a raw state. Picture the movement of your hand when you have touched red hot iron on a stove: that is the lower brain in action, jerking your hand away before you can "think" in normal Time. This awareness is a wonderful tool for a performer. In joining Time as heightened consciousness of existing in the moment, you will find an incomparable courage. A true dialogue with Time develops a sense of total independence, even from your own body. In front of an audience, facing Time, you are performing a deeply emotional and courageous act of surrender and integration with a natural force that is both inside and outside your own existence. In his recently published autobiography, Stephen Petronio writes of struggling to achieve a performance level with a new solo that Trisha Brown had just made for him:

"My experience has proven that often when a new work has its first showing for a live audience, it's only then that it rises up to become its full self. . . . I hear my introductory notes played live for the first time, I see the spiky top of Laurie Anderson's complex and beckoning head and the bow of her violin arc up in motion with a piercing sound . . . The music, the moment and the movement call me into the space I've not yet occupied and I go forth with more power than I possess. The thirty-eight seconds of motion stretch out like a bird lifting off in flight and expand to a solo of immense proportion. When I come off stage I know something has happened to me and I was prepared, lucky enough to be there and hungry enough to accept its challenge."

STEPHEN PETRONIO, Choreographer NYC
Confessions of a Motion Addict

From the Viewpoints perspective, Trisha Brown's choreography compresses Space, Shape and Time, melting one into the other. To achieve her technique one must fully embrace a fiercely articulate, fiercely kinetic movement technique.

My curiosity about Time had been fulfilled at last. Once I had experienced and experimented and established direct access to Time, I was able to be with Time through a direct connection, on my own terms. I began to understand how important it is to allow Time to be experienced, rather than counted or directed from an outside guide, even more so than the other materials of the SSTEMS. From that epiphany I found that Time and transformation are interlinked. That if we only experience numerical Time, we are prone to being frightened of and reactionary around shifts in structure. Without a true connection to Time we are much less open to possibilities. If I may say so, being in the flow of Time as it lives through your spine and connects your synapses is a much more evolved and advanced stance to inhabit in life and in art. Time, as it runs through the nervous system, is like bells ringing every moment to awaken you to a beautiful day, a beautiful life on the planet. I am wary of people with stiff spines.

In a practical application of working with Time I like to deploy a very formal Viewpoints practice. The "Viewpoints Haiku" form was invented by Wendell Beavers, a former member of my dance company, a longtime teacher at Experimental

Theatre Wing, where he taught the Viewpoints for many years, and more recently the director of the theater department at Naropa College. This form, as I use it, involves setting up a rectangle by placing shoes to mark the corners of a space approximately 9 feet by 12 feet. A group of four performers begins the form by standing in a place of their choosing on the outer edge of the rectangle. On the count of one they will all enter the space with a motion that reflects a focus on the material of Time. On the count of two they will simultaneously perform the second motion application of Time and on the count of three they will finish the haiku with a last Time-derived motion. With this, the team stops in the rectangle and then exits to restart another haiku from the periphery. The form is an interrogation instrumented by brevity, simultaneity and independence. It imparts a John Cage-like, chance operation, allowing the articulation of the material to surface with a minimum of manipulation on the part of the performer. This haiku practice is another iteration of the gesture of my hand outstretched, palm up to receive.

Using a haiku Time practice, it is immediately and thrillingly evident to observers that Time can be present in a raw form, and that Time creates fascinating performances. Just as obvious, the unilateral use of a single time signature by all performers is often boring and not necessary for building unity. Outside of traditional usage and governance, Time has the capacity to be a cohesive substance within which a fluid plethora of variations of its languages and textures can exist simultaneously.

My own dedication to the material of Time has been a bulwark of my artistic career. Underneath the minimalistic, contemplative tone of my choreography is my love for the material of Time, and the courage that this material has given me. Laurie Anderson credited me in a note on the back of her album Big Science with teaching her the concept of slow—a wisdom I seemingly imparted to her while collaborating on a music score for my choreography Hero. On this album she took seeds from her score for Hero and produced Born Never Asked.

I believe that being in contact with raw Time in as many ways as you can arrange imparts the courage to make great art. For that reason Time is also utterly present in my style of teaching. I obstinately insist on starting my classes in my own version of an American Indian type of "Gathering Time." I provide ample space for my students to arrive, and a casual conversational beginning that is designed to allow them to become present and hungry to begin work. I speak in a manner that allows thinking to occur. I wait for students to gather their thoughts. I give them more time than they need to communicate. I want them to be engaged as deeply as possible in their own reflections and responses as though they are alone in a studio working on their own ideas, in their own Time.

CHAPTER 4

Emotion

THE MATERIAL OF EMOTION IS A NATURAL PHENOMENON OF
performance. Question: what occurs when a performer stands onstage before an
audience? Answer: the performer is present. The Six Viewpoints define Emotion, at
its most basic level in performance, as the active self-awareness of the performer. I
call this self-awareness *presence*.

To begin to understand presence, the performer starts by collecting data. The
surface tension on the skin, breathing patterns, eye movements, swallowing, the
tension in the muscles of the jaw, hand movements, shifting posture, thoughts,
moods, wandering concentration, memories, concentration, wandering ideas,
avoidance or acceptance of the gaze of the audience and the feeling of acceptance
or rejection—these are all objects of careful observation. Becoming present is to
become aware of the mind and body shifting like sands in a desert.

Many performers edit out these minute details of their own state of being; it does
not occur to them to include this level of detail from themselves. This editing results
in a partial disengagement, an incomplete state of being, an abridged version of
existence. In my opinion editing the self in this way ultimately creates a less powerful
performer.

Unless gifted with presence awareness, the performer must work against a protective impulse or hiding mechanism that is triggered by lack of trust. Human instinct advises us to hide information, to avoid being fully witnessed by "the others," as a survival device in daily life. Unless a performer can establish trust in the audience and begin to dismantle their cloaking actions of "not being there" they will continue to unconsciously hide onstage. For dancers and actors the ability to release this protective mechanism allows them to draw closer to the audience and the audience to draw closer to them. In both acting and dancing, skilled presence work allows for greater visibility, since the performer is not only reaching outward but inviting the audience to come closer and watch them execute these roles as human beings.

Traditionally Emotion is handled in a noticeably different manner in dance than in theater, yet there is common ground. Let's interrogate performers' histories and then consider the training differences in emotional communication. This subject is revisited in a philosophical interrogation of the audience found in chapter 12, "The Piano: The Interface between Artist and Audience."

Traditionally in acting the playwright filters the material of Emotion through the plot of the play. In dance, this material is filtered through the physicality of the movements in the choreography. In both cases the performer must approach this task of the performance of Emotion by drawing on their own past experiences, or by focusing on evocative images.

In theater, in the 20th century, acting methodologies were formulated to achieve a realistic and truthful portrayal of Emotion in service to the play. Theater practitioners—Stanislavsky, Meyerhold, the Strasbergs, Stella Adler, Stanford Meisner, and Grotowski—all developed invaluable approaches to Emotion that are the standard of Western acting to this day.

Modern dance choreographers Martha Graham, José Limón and later Pina Bausch developed physical vocabularies into techniques designed to capture and express unique emotional content. Dancers learn to evoke Emotion through the physical techniques of the choreographers. In earlier times classical ballet dancers were taught a type of pantomime symbolizing various emotions such as love, fear and longing. As classical ballet moved into the modern era the choreographic narratives evoked animal images such as the presence of a bird (*The Firebird* choreographed by Michel Fokine with music by Stravinsky) or a faun (in *Afternoon of a Faun* choreographed by Vaslav Nijinsky with music by Debussy).

A performer who has mastered the material of Emotion, from the perspective of the SSTEMS interrogation of the Six Viewpoints, has the ability to exist fully onstage under the gaze of the audience, communicating human to human. This total interface between the performer and their audience is what I label presence. Rather than replacing traditional approaches to emotion, presence can provide a fascinating basis. To be present in your own breathing, sensing, thinking, seeing, hearing and processing is for some performers natural and a part of their acting technique; for others this stance can be more difficult. In either situation, investigating Emotion as presence invites a poetic view of the discipline of performance and can be enormously helpful as an artistic tool.

The technique of presence reminds me of the Zen koan. Both are minimal, elegant and yet contain so much in such a small act. Powerful aspects of performance, being in contact with a microscopic awareness of yourself and how you are received that is often hidden by conventional acting and dancing, can surface when Emotion is reduced to presence. This "koan" begins with placing the performer onstage without anything, narrative or choreographic, to perform.

Presence essentially changes the game plan of most performance training. The ability to perform your own presence is essential for the performer in establishing a wide and grounded understanding of the natural basis of communication in the theater. Through the Viewpoints presence training the performers discover not only themselves but also better understand the audience.

Here is how, based on my observations, to begin building an awareness of the performer's more expanded self, eventually leading to a greater command of presence. First, have the performer sit in front of a class, with nothing to perform, and collect data about themselves as they consciously allow themselves to be watched. A narrative of this activity might look like this:

Ahh, here I am and they are watching me. This is causing my breathing to be fairly shallow, there is a rigidity in my body and especially in my spine; I don't feel comfortable with them watching me; now a wave of sensation is rippling up the surface of my back; I am acutely aware of my shoulders for some reason; I need to allow them to see that I am uncomfortable. My focus could be more acute; I am in a mild fog. I would like to swallow and instead grind my teeth lightly; they can see me grinding my teeth. I have stopped breathing for a second. I shift my ribcage and take a deep breath that moves my last three ribs. I just dropped my eyelids; I am going to keep them down and let myself know that they can see this gesture, this action, the vulnerable position. I look up, smile nervously at my audience, taking a ragged breath. This is my current state of being.

As performers bringing this version of themselves to life, they must occasionally dare to look directly into the eyes of their audience. This act assures that they are not avoiding any aspect of acknowledgment that they are there before a witness. If all is going well, the performer will accumulate the ability to be *present* and gain a thrilling experience: the gift of being seen. It is important to note that in order to perform this practice you must try to embrace the idea that you are loved and allowed to sit there. Some performers can actually feel that they are not wanted onstage.

It is important to note that things can go wrong in the practice. To avoid the task of being present students will sometimes resort to faux realistic activities such as pulling at their clothes or fixating on a button. These make-believe activities usually enter into a continuous rhythm that keeps the student distracted from the reality of being before our eyes. When these behaviors are observed the teacher must remind the student to refocus on what is being seen, on what is present in themselves.

In an effort to introduce Emotion as presence to students at the Experimental Theatre Wing, I began calling the practice the Dog-Sniff-Dog World. Pure presence is a shared instinct, easier to observe in dogs but still always there in every meeting of human with human as well. We are all capable of reading through presence the countless indicators of state of mind and emotional condition. I think New Yorkers enjoy engaging in this under the protection of the semi-anonymity of streets and subways. To demonstrate this Dog-Sniff-Dog World I suggest to my students that we could bring someone in from the street and have them simply stand in our studio for three minutes; upon their exit the class defines their state of mental and physical health and articulates the major traits of their personality. This instinctual ability is ingrained in us. We only block it because we are wary of getting caught or being placed in a dangerous situation. I think performers should interrogate their own presence, and by doing this they become independent performing artists capable of approaching the audience directly and with great subtlety.

When you are able to experience and perform presence on the level of the Six Viewpoints you will find a new meaning and understanding of what can and does transpire in performance.

All of my favorite performers and directors have a clear grasp of presence, whether it is in their own performance or in the content of composition, from Dolly Parton to Robert Wilson, from Johnny Depp to Yvonne Rainer, from Richard Foreman to Philip Glass. In my view the specific content and esthetic does not truly matter. This direct contact with the audience, along with the clarity of what is being delivered, gives the performer an exquisite feeling of being included in communication with the audience.

In several of my early dances, *Adam* and *Painters Dream* for instance, I explored the element of presence as one of the main experimental focuses.

In *Adam* I decided to make a solo about my father Olav. I am not a biographer or a portrait artist. I used him to study how he used presence. He rarely spoke yet was in constant communication with all around him. As a farmer, surveyor and lover of nature he was emotionally present with nature. I thought that if I made a theater piece based on his presence, I would have a unique opportunity to study a nonverbal state of Emotion.

I structured this solo as a kind of haiku, paring down the physical staging to the bare necessities. This seemed appropriate to his way of being and to the possibility of examining Emotion under a high-powered microscope. The solo contained the following elements: lying on a mattress in three positions, sitting in one position, walking five steps forward on a diagonal, standing, walking five steps back, and repeating these movements in any order with any timing for 20 minutes. The experiment was to see if the audience could read, through my presence, my thoughts and emotions, as I had read those of my father many years ago.

The solo became a cornerstone of my research into Emotion. Through this work I learned how to relax in front of an audience, to allow them to read me, and to refrain from covering my fear of being watched by being entertaining. The audience reported that they found the performance a highly emotional experience. They felt that they could read my thoughts. They could read me! This solo eventually formed the basis of the presence practice that is now part of the Viewpoints classroom.

When an actor or a dancer comes to stand as an equal observer/participant with this material of Emotion through presence, they can start to perceive how accurately, in the emotional world, people can read the presence of other people and establish a performance that fully converses with the audience.

In this presence practice, the performer begins to grow in performative and conceptual substance. Over the span of a semester I watch as this experience of presence grows and takes hold in students' concept of what can happen in the theater. They feel increasingly at home and welcomed having tested the waters of their own presence. A fragile but powerful performer emerges: the uncloaked human being! Through the interrogation of their natural presence the performer can experience the thrill of being fully present in front of the audience.

CHAPTER 5

Movement

IN INTERROGATING THE MATERIAL OF MOVEMENT, THE VIEWPOINTS once again look beyond the established systems of magnificent techniques that have been codified into training methods. The goal here is to discuss the essential nature of Movement so that the performer may have a one-on-one dialogue with it. We are seeking the absolute core in order to define this material that lies so close to the bone. The interrogation:

The core nature of dance is Movement.

The core nature of Movement resides in our ability to experience kinetic sensation.

Beginning with a deconstructive, pre-movement/natural approach, in which the performer is able to read and generate kinetic sensation, we can interrogate Movement to begin to build a physical dialogue free of cultured confines. This may seem like a very internal, almost anti-performance, but on this level dance and theater are fully connected. And with the rather recent discovery of mirror neurons, we know that the brain of the observer is stimulated in exactly the same manner as the person performing a movement. Neural interconnectivity between performer and viewer functions as a profound element of both acting and dancing. The kinetic sensation of a fall is felt by all.

Stripped of Shape, Space, Time, and Emotion, Movement still contains a world of infinitely subtle communication.

I first witnessed the direct tie to Movement as kinetic sensation while attending the performances of Grand Union, the improvisation performance group initiated by Yvonne Rainer. She concocted kinetic situations, such as running with a mattress held between all the performers in a full-out celebration of kinetic sensation. In a later performance, a member of Grand Union, Steve Paxton (the inventor of Contact Improvisation) decided not to move a muscle for the duration of a performance. Standing in complete apparent stillness, in the absence of movement, the kinetics of this material oozed throughout the entire performance. asserting its power and place in the SSTEMS.

This seventies, SoHo view of movement as kinetic sensation helped performers get past "the performing bear world," as innovator Yvonne Rainer once condemned traditional dance in Time magazine. She wanted to do away with the confining definition of dance as a type of physical/artistic sport. Rainer deplored the idea of dance defined by how high dancers could lift their leg, spin or jump. She rightly realized that these "requirements" reduced the art form to something close to a carnival show. Her inclusion of pedestrian movement as dance flipped the genre upside down and allowed it to fully enter the art world. She reduced dance to its essence of kinetic sensation, and this separation from traditional technique allowed every dancer to be an artist in possession of their own medium. The impact of including walking in her dance vocabulary, encouraged individual dancers/artists to use the materials (Space, Shape, Time, Emotion, Movement and Logic) to serve their own means. In my opinion, this embrace of the materials set in motion a revolutionary and lasting contribution to dance.

In this new interpretation of dance, dancers themselves decided what materials they worked with, no longer obligated to use an arabesque in every performance to prove they were indeed performing dance. Dance can now include falling, rolling or crawling and the performance of these kinetic motions requires a different type of physical training. Different techniques came to satisfy this need—Alexander Technique, Kinetic Awareness, Body-Mind Centering and Feldenkrais Method, to name just a few of the more well known training methods. Physical training on this level develops a direct connection to the forces affecting our bodies internally and externally, and as a result the performer's movement articulation is enhanced.

During the sixties and seventies, dance artists stopped studying the body through traditional techniques and went straight to the body itself. This is the "rolling on the floor generation," taking the body out of its formal dance training systems and deconstructing movement through anatomical study and improvisation. Steve Paxton's Contact Improvisation is one of the best examples of this type of new training methodology. This is a method of movement generation based on two bodies using one point of balance. His work is invaluable to both actors and dancers because it achieves a familiarity with kinetic motion that interfaces directly with the physical sensation, breaks the formal social barriers between bodies and carries the understanding of movement into a universal, deeply natural realm.

In this environment I came to the conclusion that to be at the fundamental source of Movement you must study motion as sensation. Like me, many young dance artists had individual, laboratory-like studios. These laboratories sprang up throughout SoHo. Each contained its own wizard/alchemist, with their experimentations and new perspectives. This changing approach to Movement influenced not only the training and repertoire of dancers, but spilled over into the way contemporary actors were, and are, trained. Suddenly everyone, theater artists and dancers alike, was concerned with locating the sensation of the spine, the ability to roll and return to standing with efficiency, etc. I regard this sensual movement training as reflecting the beginning of an explosion in human physical achievements that also ran through the sports world, developing into extreme skiing and hang gliding, and bursting out into the street as breakdancing and hip hop.

You can see this quality of Movement and physical sensation in the work of actor Willem Dafoe. In plays such as The Hairy Ape, directed by Elizabeth LeCompte, his physical kinetic movement onstage almost obliterates the rest of the SSTEMS. Space, blocking, timing, line delivery, the visuals of the set and even the story are left clinging and fighting for dear life, threatened by the raw presence of Movement. Another example is the sensuous movement of the Pina Bausch Company in choreographies such as her Café Mueller. Here the performers present a heightened visceral iteration of dance. You feel you are breathing with them rather than simply watching them. Their ability to communicate directly through kinetic sensation casts that energy right into the audience. Our mirror neurons are dazzled. Every performance they give is experienced as a hyper-kinetic event. A performer who has a full awareness of the kinetic sensation of movement can communicate this quality even in stillness. When a dancer or actor who is aware of sensation merely stands, you feel their muscles ripple and sense their blood, warm and fluid.

In the Six Viewpoints approach, to truly come into its own, Movement must be removed from form constraints. As a practice method I return to the haiku form, using Movement as the material so that my students can experience and witness pure kinetics at work without any preset forms or interference from exteriorized Time or Shape. Eliminating those two design elements/materials, a body moves from pure sensation, and is a transcendent joy to watch. Movement stripped away from the other artful languages allow the students to see its impact and carry it into performance with confidence in its raw beautiful quality.

Much physical training precedes this haiku practice. To enter the material of Movement, students must learn falling, rolling, standing and walking until they find the kinetic core of their movement. If you want to be a strong and independent performer, you alone must reclaim your physical identity, stolen from you by social restrictions on Movement. You must remove the blocks that stifle physical contact with others, cause the fear of falling and the shame of physical sensation in general. In the end, just as with the other SSTEMS, kinetic sensation must be discovered as a one- on-one dialogue. As all great movement performers know, you must fight all barriers to sensation. You must conquer these limitations inside your own body. Finally, you must get past formal exterior movement training in order to own your movement.

Much of my exploration into movement training for actors took place in the studios of the Experimental Theatre Wing (ETW) at New York University. At the core of this training program I applied this concept of movement through sensation via a technique I call the Hamilton Floor Barre. This system was invented by Jean

Hamilton, who deconstructed ballet to find what could help students who were of attention paid to the functioning of the joints and articulation of the body in alignment—an astonishing amount of knowledge contained in directional intentions of movement resulting in performative strength and control. Toward the middle of my classes at ETW, in the third or fourth week of study, I pair this training with Contact Improvisation to round out the student's sensory radar. I believe that these two training components impart an acute ability in students to create their onstage actions from sensation rather than from exterior/learned/repetitive systems such as those taught in modern dance or the martial arts.

The responsibility we shouldered in those early days at ETW was staggering and thrilling. Our faculty meetings were absolute shirtsleeves-rolled-up work sessions. There was to be no hierarchy in the training. We would coexist and contribute our techniques and experiments to one "pot." This pot would be the students; no one would own or dominate. The students' growth would be our goal. No one was even tempted to use the studio to build an unchallengeable domination, an exclusive leadership. No one was right and no one was wrong. I first encountered the Grotowski Plastiques there, with the horizontal experimental environment of the 1978 art world raging just outside our doors. The Plastiques and the Viewpoints became the natural foundation for the school at a very early stage of development. Through this combination the movement and acting faculty brought kinetic sensation to the table.

Of course this coexistence was not always comfortable. I was irritated by the Grotowski training because I felt that the Plastiques were unnecessarily stressful on the body. They did not provide enough visceral anatomical information, such as alignment training, proper stretches, and careful joint strengthening. From my own postmodern perspective on Movement, these Grotowski neighbors were loud, frenetic, stressed, narrow, mindless, and lacking subtlety. In comparison to the Plastiques, my classes had the atmosphere of a Buddhist temple. In the end I came to appreciate the viability of the Grotowski work as invaluable acting/physical training and found it amusing how well these two forms fit together in the end. Since that faraway time, two very advanced forms of actor training have evolved that, in the capable hands of brilliant actors/directors Erica Fay and Rainer Von Walden, who combine Viewpoints and Grotowski.

As a child I devoted myself to running up and down hills, bicycling, mountain climbing, balancing on anything precarious—conducting an interrogation of the earth's forces in a celebration and love of my muscles. To this day I tend to be a muscle-centric dancer. At nine I understood that dance would be my profession. I cannot recall how I got to this determination since I had not seen any dance. Perhaps it was my attachment to Greek mythology and the stories of the bull dancers. I began studying ballet at Robert DeWeese's painting studio.

A former dancer, Harvey Jung had returned to Montana to attend Montana State University in Bozeman and fallen in with the DeWeese art circle. Longing to be near dance he asked permission to teach at Bob's studio. He had attempted to choreograph after years of performing as a child star and later as a company member of the Metropolitan Opera Ballet in New York. His creative efforts caused him to have a nervous breakdown and he was in the process of redirecting his life by going back to school. I joined four other students in his classes, which were strictly conducted and did not include any learned movement beyond the ballet barre. He had concluded that it was all that learned movement that had caused him to be inhibited as a creative spirit. I thought that improvisation and ballet barre was "ballet" until, at 14, when I received a scholarship to spend one summer studying at Cranbrook College, "back east", in Michigan. I took a real ballet class and when they started center floor I was amazed at how everyone was doing the same movements. I kept bumping into dancers until I retreated to the corner.

Even with the terrifying concept that dance was based on learning movements that were performed in groups, I nonetheless ran away from home. I was 17 years old with 50 dollars in my pocket, hopping freight trains to get to "the dance." Nothing could slow the urge and thrill of my love of sensation and my commitment to the vocabulary of communication through movement. I pursued more ballet, then modern, then Cunningham and finally postmodern, improvisation, Contact Improvisation and a plethora of alternative studies of the body. I retooled my body yet again at age 30 with ballet training from a system invented and taught by Jean Hamilton (who danced with

Pavlova on the South American tour), then choreographed more and trained other dancers and actors. This is my family: the dancers, the kinetic artists.

CHAPTER 6

Story

As human beings we reflexively and successfully sort tons of information on a daily basis, formulating a living ongoing story. This material, interrogated as a natural phenomenon, turns into particles that turn into an arrangement of those particles, exposing the manipulation of logic that is the core of Story. Story in the Six Viewpoints is simply seen as a specific logic that functions as an organization of sequences of information. For innovative artists, the material of Story/Logic is often the most challenging and difficult topic to deal with.

Interrogating Story as Logic, the material becomes easily identifiable as integral to both theatrical story and choreography. Seen as Logic, Story also seamlessly unites two important voices in art often viewed as opposite, those of abstraction and those of realism. At the heart of both are specific arrangements of Story/Logic. This essential material is found at work in all languages and art: words, numbers, music, movement, painting, carpentry, architecture, engineering, the sciences.

Linking Story with Logic facilitates a more open dialogue with performance. I will explain later in this chapter why I use the word Story in the SSTEMS rather than Logic, but for now I am asking you to accept the two labels as interchangeable in the Viewpoints system.

To examine this material fully I like to begin by focusing on what keeps the whole structure of Story/Logic on track, its primal function in life. Without the ability to use this tool we would have perished long ago. This is what gives this material its edgy quality in all the arts. Artists who master this material will consequently create a voice heard by their generation, and may even shape the future development of dance and theater. While it is possible to direct and choreograph being only semi-conscious of this material, your work will be pale and have little impact. If you are sensitive to how Logic is wired into our instincts, you will challenge yourself to struggle for maximum clarity within the sequences and languages of your work.

I like to think about art in this way because it reminds me that art must grapple with communication. By acknowledging that we are natural and obsessive sleuths ("What was that sound?" "How did the cat get in the house?" "Why is that person looking at me that way?" "Is this good to eat or will it poison me?") we can grasp this essential component of the creative process.

Focusing on Story/Logic as a guiding principle, theater and dance makers are constantly exposed to the challenge of a maddeningly sensitive material whose primary characteristic is mutability. Story/Logic confronts the artist with the necessity of establishing and understanding their own set of principles, rules and esthetics. Just as with the other SSTEMS, Logic is the artist's constant companion. How much you want to embrace it depends on your courage and dedication.

For the performer, Logic is key to understanding the intent of the director/choreographer. The performer shoulders the responsibility of communicating the "message." Most successful artists are hyperaware that the clarity of the "logic" behind a work will determine how well the art will be received. In my opinion, if art fails to impress, it is because the artist and or the performer has failed to accurately present a clear and engaging Logic.

Many audiences do not understand that this material costs the artist much time and anguish. The audience who is appreciative of this struggle derives greater pleasure out of art. In any given moment of a performance, there are infinite options for where an actor or dancer is physically placed but only one position will express the Logic of a particular work. The establishment of place may take enormous time to ascertain and even then may need to be reconfigured when a new set of blocking or choreography is added. This feature of Story/Logic is the most difficult of the SSTEMS to teach since it is so intrinsic to personal vision and esthetic.

The invisible and often frustrating work that goes into establishing the Story/Logic of a creative piece lacks the glamour of working with Space, Shape, Time, Emotion or Movement since it is totally intangible. But in my opinion this struggle is also thrillingly complex and rewarding beyond the other SSTEMS.

I must divulge how I came to use the term Story in my theory, since I honestly prefer the term Logic. In my era of Conceptual Minimalism, Merce Cunningham, John Cage and many of my colleagues made broad public statements that their work had nothing to do with Story. Composer John Cage loved to find methods that would allow two sounds to be placed next to each other without his having chosen what their placement was. These careful, rigorous and sometimes agonizingly time-consuming processes removed any chance that he had built a story into his work. Story in his eyes represented a lesser concept than the incidents or accidents that occur in the universe surrounding us. Artists like Cage scoffed at the old-fashioned and confining forms of Story. These artists were trying to get the audience to pay attention to a larger sphere. They were staging an all-out attack on the dominating and hierarchical position of Story in performing arts. In defending and staking out their territory their statement was: THIS DOES NOT MEAN ANYTHING. This statement was, and is meant, to redirect our attention to a vast array of sounds, logics, structures, spaces, movements, shapes, times, dimensions.

But I disagreed. Although I identify as being part of this generation of work, I felt and still feel that their pronouncements, however revolutionary, were dangerous in ways they were not seeing. The power of Story is so important to human communication that to divorce this material from the magnificent work they were doing caused their message to be somewhat misunderstood. THEIR WORK DID MEAN SOMETHING and did have a Story, just not the traditional Story. Its Story was that we can read Logic in so many different ways. So to challenge them, I used the term Story when Logic would have been far more acceptable and accurate to the thinking of my generation, especially when I was making a deconstruction of theater and dance.

No one made any objection, because I did not state my opinions on "No Story" back then. If I had, I probably would have been dismissed as ignorant, for I was surrounded by artists who were restructuring the notion of Story in their art. Richard Serra, Richard Nonas, Keith Sonnier, Dan Flavin and Donald Judd were making non-object sculptures; Philip Glass, Terry Riley and Ornette Coleman were making non-symphonic symphonies; Joan Jonas and Patti Smith were making non-performance performance; Richard Foreman, Lee Breuer, Joanne Akalitis and Liz LeCompte were making non-narrative theater and Lucinda Childs, Steve Paxton, Yvonne Rainer, Barbara Dilley and Robert Dunn were making non-dance dances. They were introducing new Logic and were very convincing in their interrogative skill and passion, I followed everything they did in awe.

Putting my art on the line I insisted that there was Story in abstraction. Many of my early choreographies were inspired by an artistic dialogue I was having with Merce Cunningham under the category "Arguments with Merce." These works were what I came to call "Abstract Narratives." I agree that Merce's work has no traditional narrative logic (which is very hard to do given that we are all natural questioners, searching for answers), but his enormous effort to have no Story is itself the Logic.

My first Abstract Narratives worked with choreography that was based on the space where the dance would be performed. Window Pieces was a three-year series constructed for, and performed in, the windows of the Holly Solomon Gallery on West Broadway, from 1976 to 1979. This project was followed by Painters Dream and Hero at the Kitchen Center for Video, Music and Dance when it was located on Grand Street. In these narratives, Space, Shape, Time, Movement, and Emotion/ Presence were woven together in a carefully chosen sequential structure based on the architecture. The experiments in these dances became my springboard into the art world, resulting in an invitation to help start the Experimental Theatre Wing at NYU. Regular performances in Europe and many years of happily performing and instructing young theater artists and dancers around the world followed.

Through the lens of Logic, we can trace different manipulations of Story versus non-Story within the world of playwriting. Traditional playwrights create stories in additive sequential logic. Family connections are often important and consistent throughout the play and give reference points for the audience through which to see the actions evolve. Tensions are introduced and result in explosions of confrontation and find various resolutions at the end of the performance. Emotions are carefully drawn to support the Story, as are the blocking, the timing, the movement, and the gestures of the actors.

I tend to like the playwrights who work in a more horizontal, nonhierarchical basis: Maria Irene Fornés, Sam Shepard, and Samuel Beckett, to name a few. These playwrights do not necessarily set their stories in "real" worlds, and the events that transpire often CANNOT be understood in terms of traditional Story form (beginning, middle and end). When we watch a play by Irene Fornés, her situations, characters, costumes, and dialogue are odd companions. Nothing seems to be created to fit together. But this jagged juxtaposition is what generates the energy and empathy, humor and horror, of her Story. We are brought down from some clean, lofty, superior, organized place of traditional Story to wallow in the mud and then emerge to find ourselves floating in waters of beneficent forgiveness and acceptance.

I am a much better person after watching these playwrights' work because I have been taught to see the world with more complex appreciation through their masterful manipulation of Logic. They painstakingly represent a real world where judgment and certainty is absurd. This is the vast and powerful territory of Story/Logic: I am socially and politically a more evolved human being from watching their plays. Logic is their tool and we are the beneficiaries of their efforts.

Lee Breuer's intricate biography of his father, who is portrayed as a workhorse in Red Horse Animations, is full of love and wonder at life. What comes across the stage in shapes, space, movement, sound and timing is the articulation of a logic in which the monotony of his father's work is slowly killing him. Breuer's signature Logic is tidal and circular. As with all good or great art, every moment of Breuer's work is crisp and clean with intention, yet the Story/Logic flows back and forth, from now to the past, from space to the presence of the performers. It ripples with emotions that are as chaotic as life or landscape.

When the SSTEMS as employed as discrete elements of the natural stage, the material of Story/Logic has a wider palette and venue. In my opinion, dance is often weak when it comes to well thought-out and intricate use of Logic. Perhaps this is because it does not directly tell stories through words, and the subject of the work gets left out or is a very small consideration. I encourage young choreographers to study Logic as it stands naked onstage, that is, as an art form not based in the human "story" but stripped naked in a deeply involved and engaged union with all of the SSTEMS. At the Experimental Theatre Wing, we require a good helping of dance solos to give young actors and directors the chance to strengthen their structural/ Logic abilities without the use of words.

Choreographers construct dances out of the materials of Space, Shape, Time and Movement; all of which require logical choices. But often they fail to find a unique separate logical statement that stands apart from their moment-to-moment work with the materials. Too often the overall structural integrity of the choreography is weak. Dance, similar to traditional theater's desire for conflict, traditionally focuses on the demands of kinetics to dictate to Logic. But if Logic is engaged as a separate material the possibility for more profound meaning is enhanced.

An example of an intricate and unblemished manipulation of Logic can be found in the choreographies of Lucinda Childs. There is minimal movement vocabulary— running, skipping and small leaps—yet the monotonous flow of Time, as expressed in massive spatial patterns, provides structure. Her exploitation of the power of Story/Logic delivers a pleasure as immense as watching a ballet dancer leap to great heights, but a pleasure that is richer because it stimulates the mind.

While the flow of Logic is one aspect of Story/Logic, another is what I call arcing. Here I refer to a mechanism seen in the tungsten light bulb. In the light bulb, electricity jumps/arcs between two separate wires, thereby emitting light. Working with my students to further liberate the material of Logic, I encourage them to experiment with Story in horizontal conditions similar to that of the light bulb. Arcing happens in performance when information of any kind, such as actions, objects, timing, or words, are placed next to each other. The artist allows them to remain next to each other until they begin to emit Logic. These elements begin to "spark" off each other and meaning starts to shine through. The information or Story/Logic that results is far more interesting than anything you could just think up. You will find in the Practice Manual an exercise dealing with this principle. As it plays in a no man's land of absolute chance operation and new logics, this exercise, The Fifth Story, transports the observer/performer to another world of Story that is beyond the manipulation of Logic. Stories, normally made accessible by our habitual grasping for the security of hierarchically organized meaning, get rerouted, adding greater complexity and more subtle meaning.

Now consider Story in a different iteration. We're going to address the Story/Logic of black-dot-on-a-white-canvas art. Over the centuries there have been many battles between the concepts of realism and abstraction. How can abstract art communicate anything? What is it about? During the 20th century, these were common questions hurled at the "new" art form of abstraction. Another was whether this art requires any skill, although the "my monkey could do that" reaction has somewhat receded. I feel that the reason that such art is readable and valuable is still not well understood. In order to make strong abstract work it is critical to fathom the logic of your choices and the history and context of those choices. I compare this to a lone mountain climber gazing up at the face of a sheer granite wall. The route he or she plots out could mean life or death, success or failure. I find that abstract art that is "soft" on the issues of Logic very often falls into a type of reflexive faux abstraction. and that contemporary art that employs realism often ends up making unexamined bows to abstraction. In the absence of logical decisions early on, such art finds itself on a trajectory to mediocrity. Early in the process of a new abstract work, when your impulses are riding high, the search for the rationale, the Logic, is creative and thrilling.

We can use the Viewpoints to begin to understand abstract art and its impact it on society. A white canvas with a black dot is dealing with logic. If the dot is centered, it has a different impact on us than if it were placed in any of the millions of other possible positions. We read where the fire hydrant is placed and do not run into it on the way to the subway. We care about this reading with a spatial passion and with this same logic we care where that black dot is placed. Why we care is linked with the way we care about our orbiting pattern in relationship to the sun. We feel it with our bodies, we see it with our eyes, and we respond to it in our lives. Abstract art manifests its logic through the universal languages of Space, Time, Shape, Emotion, Movement, and Story. The manipulation of logic in abstract art places the audience outside their daily lives, connecting them to the drama of existence.

In my fascination with and effort to impart the importance of Logic to my students, I trace over the obvious again. The material of Story exists because of our ability to gather, relate, deduce and draw conclusions from information. If you want to make great art you must create great logic.

The replacement of one "fact" with another can shift the logical outcome of a story to devastating or enlightening effects. The world is still intrigued by the creation of Michelangelo's David. The solitary figure evokes endless adoration. This has been explained, in part, by the fact that David's hand is not in proportion to the rest of his body. And yet, in its unrealistic dimension, it balances the entire structure and allows the eye to flow over the figure. This manipulation of logic makes this sculpture resonate and inspire. Logic is essential to art, in every medium.

What are the sources of Logic? How do you deal with this material in such a way that it remains alive and vital in the viewer's experience? In my introductory lecture on the Six Viewpoints I stand and hold my hand out from my body, palm cupped toward the ceiling and say, "See this? This is the Six Viewpoints." Then I stare at my hand for a moment. Without taking my eyes off my hand I say. "At any moment this is going to become a performance, it is going to become art . . . it's going to start to take on a meaning, a story." At first it seems like a joke. But before even one ripple of laughter can rise, what I am saying sinks in. As the meaning arrives everyone does manage to laugh. But it is a very different kind of laughter than derision. It is the laugh of a sudden realization. Art can only happen if you have the sensibility to perceive it.

To begin to approach the world of Story/Logic wearing artist's glasses, I have students improvise on the topics of a refrigerator, a white wall, a coat-hanger, or a wastebasket. These seemingly bland, undramatic, if not totally irrelevant topics appear at first to be dry wells as sources. How could any of them even have a Story? I tell them to pay no attention to their misgivings or judgments. I ask them to just try this practice out with a shrug, indicating that this is a very inconsequential practice. Once they begin, they are astonished at the number of Stories these things contain. Through this practice I approach Story from a tricky back door. If something that seems this banal has stories, then Story must exist everywhere. The students begin looking with shining eyes, artist's eyes, hungry for all the stories that must be tucked away, hiding in the shadow of the monolithic traditional idea of Story.

The material of Story/Logic has been a bright thread running through my own creative work, my teaching and my views of the world of art. In constructing your own work and especially when making less traditional, more abstract work, it is not easy to remember the critical importance of the manipulation of Logic. Of all the SSTEMS, even beyond the striking effect that "discovery" of Space and the profound impact of presence have on my students, it is Story/Logic that is the material I most want my students to understand and master.

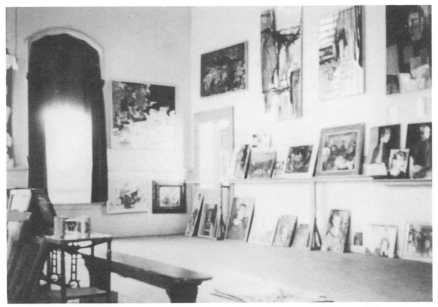

Bob DeWeese Studio circa 1956. On the far wall is the ballet barre installed for Overlie's teacher Harvey Jung's dance class.

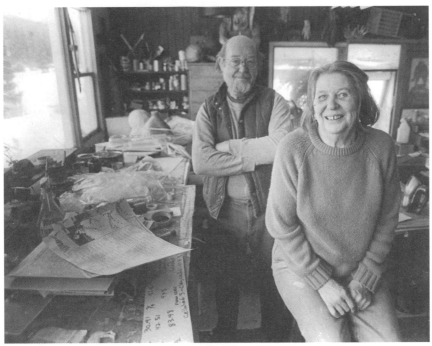

Bob and Gennie DeWeese in Gennie's studio at their home, Bozeman, Montana circa 1980s.

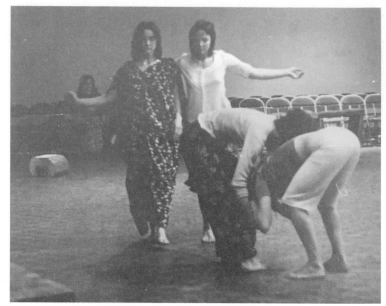

Natural History of the American Dancer Lesser Known Species, Volume 12 thru 24, Whitney Museum of American Art concert, 1972. Left to right: Carmen Beuchat, Barbara Dilley, Suzanne Harris, Cynthia Hedstrom, Mary Overlie, Judy Padow, Rachael Wood.

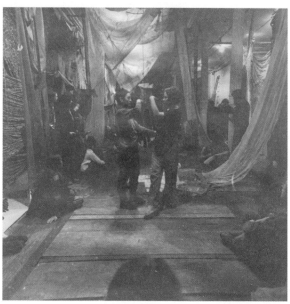

Natural History of the American Dancer, 112 Greene Street Gallery, 1972. Left to right: Carmen Beuchat, Barbara Dilley, with Yvonne Rainer in the audience. Photographer: Randal Arabie.

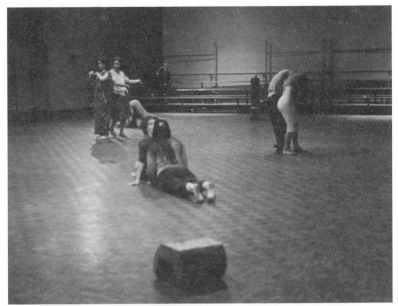

Natural History of the American Dancer Lesser Known Species; volume 12 thru 24 Whitney Museum concert, 1972. Left to right: Carmen Beuchat, Barbara Dilley, Mary Overlie, Judy Padow.

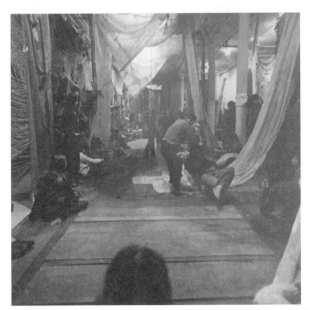

Natural History of the American Dancer, 112 Greene Street Gallery, 1972. Left to right: Carmen Beuchat, Barbara Dilley, Suzanne Harris and Cynthia in background, with Yvonne Rainer in the audience. Photographer: Randal Arabie.

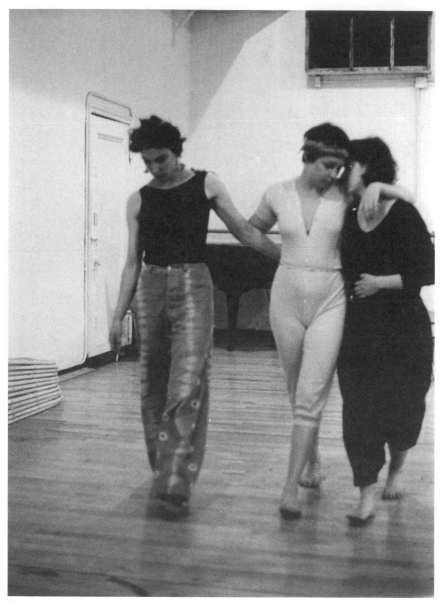

Natural History of the American Dancer, Larry Richardson Dance Gallery, 1974. Left to right: Mary Overlie, Barbara Dilley, Cynthia Hedstrom.

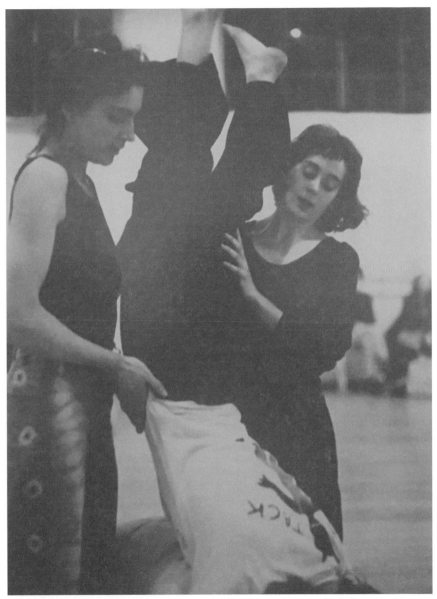

Natural History of the American Dancer, Larry Richardson Dance Gallery ,1974. Left to right: Mary Overlie, Cynthia Hedstrom, Judy Padow.

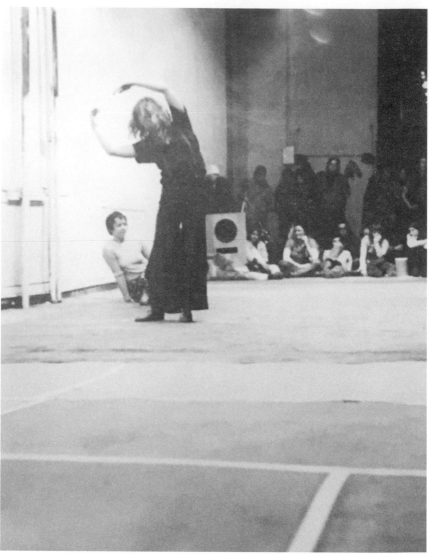

Natural History of the American Dancer, 112 Greene Street Gallery, 1972. Left to right: Barbara Dilley, Suzanne Harris.

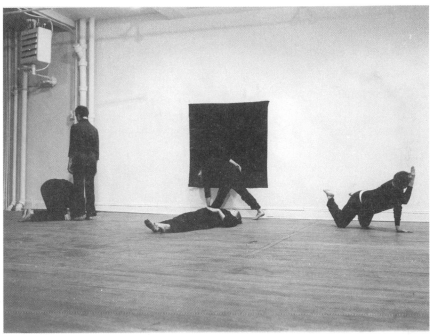

Natural History of the American Dancer, Paula Cooper Gallery, 1975. Left to right: Carmen Beuchat, Suzanne Harris, Cynthia Hedstrom, Mary Overlie, Rachael Wood.

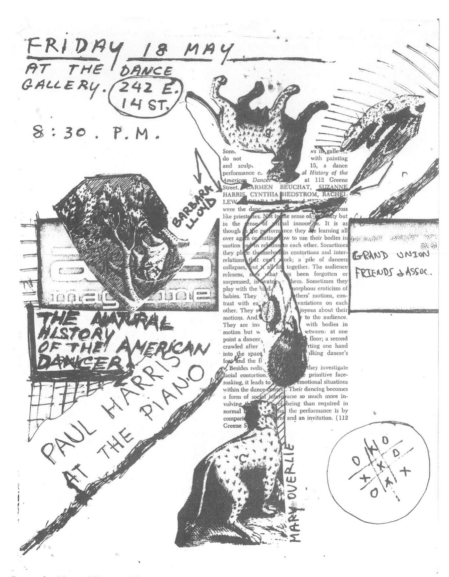

Poster for *Natural History of the American Dancer*, Paula Cooper Gallery, 1973.

BY ROSEMARY MAYER

Some of the more successful shows in galleries
do not necessarily deal solely with painting
and sculpture. On October 15, a dance
performance called the *Natural History of the
American Dancer* unfolded at 112 Greene
Street. CARMEN BEUCHAT, SUZANNE
HARRIS, CYNTHIA HEDSTROM, RACHEL
LEW, BARBARA LLOYD, and JUDY PADOW
were the dancers/performers who come across
like priestesses. Not in the sense of solemnity but
in the sense of primal innocence. It is as
though in the performance they are learning all
over again or testing how to use their bodies in
motion and in relation to each other. Sometimes
they place themselves in contortions and inter-
relations that can't work; a pile of dancers
collapses, but it all fits together. The audience
relearns, sees what has been forgotten or
surpressed, in watching them. Sometimes they
play with the kind of polymorphous eroticism of
babies. They mimic each others' motions, contrast with each other, do variations on each
other. They seem absolutely joyous about their
motions. And that comes over to the audience.
They are involved not only with bodies in
motion but with the spaces between: at one
point a dancer walked across the floor; a second
crawled after her carefully inserting one hand
into the space between the walking dancer's
foot and the floor.

Besides rediscovering motion they investigate
facial contortions. Initially like primitive face-
making, it leads to personal, emotional situations
within the dance context. Their dancing becomes
a form of social intercourse so much more in-
volving the totality of being than required in
normal interactions that the performance is by
comparision a comment and an invitation. (112
Greene St. *Oct. 15.*)

DECEMBER JANUARY 1973

Arts Magazine review, January 1973, *Natural History of the American Dancer,* Paula Cooper Gallery.
Performers: Carmen Beuchat, Suzanne Harris, Cynthia Hedstrom, Mary Overlie, Rachael Wood.

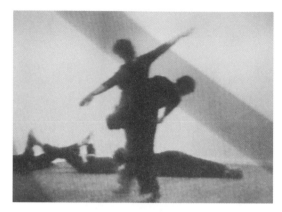

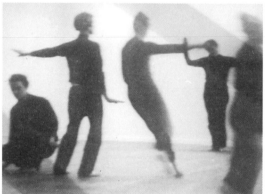

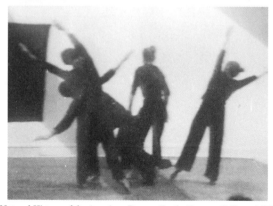

Natural History of the American Dancer, Paula Cooper Gallery, 1975.

COMMENTS FROM OTHER ARTISTS

While shooting video tape of this group of dancers I felt powerfully drawn by the group's centering psychic energy. Interaction of human presences; communication of brains. If the space-time continuum can become an esthetic experience, this is them, spiraling and circling, sharing their personal spaces, breaking apart and reweaving themselves. Intangible network. Real invisible web. Build-up toward harmony. Breaking loose. Regerminating. The natural muscle is transcended into an abstraction of human relations.

Jaun Downey painter and video artist

The work is open and fresh. Dealing with the weight of the body in relation to the floor and in relation to eachother draws the spectator into the energy of the performance. Afterwards I want to dance.

Joan Jonas dancer and choreographer

When you watch the Natural History move it is like a secret between you - them and you. Everyone has a different secret with the Natural History, mine is that I'm watching the movement of their minds and the information that I get is very personal - and it is true.

Lee Brewer writer and director of Mabu Mines

The Natural History of the American Dancer are a unique group of dancers. Bond together by a poetry of movement, they display through their various abilities the roots of dance. Theirs is an evolution of movement, the place and time of gesture and consciousness of expanding limits as well as frailties. Dance for them becomes an exorcism.

Allen Katzman poet

Arts Magazine review, January 1973, *Natural History of the American Dancer,* Paula Cooper Gallery. Comments from other artists, including Juan Downey, Joan Jonas, Lee Breuer and Allen Katzman.

PART TWO

THE
BRIDGE

The Nine Laboratories of the Bridge

News of a Difference
Noticing Difference in Increasing
Levels of Subtlety

Deconstruction
Investigating Theater by Separating
the Components of Its Structure

The Horizontal
Nonhierarchical Composition

Postmodernism
The Philosophical Foundation

Reification
A Reflection on Creativity,
Communication, and Language

The Piano
The Interface between Artist and Audience

The Matrix
The Ingredients Are in the Cauldron

Doing the Unnecessary
The SSTEMS Dissolve

The Original Anarchist
A New and Very Old Idea

INTRODUCTION

The Bridge

THE BRIDGE, CONTAINING NINE LABORATORIES, PRESENTS THE ORIGINS of the Viewpoints' approach to art. These laboratories focus attention on philosophical concepts that are used to disintegrate and then reintegrate performance. In order to explain this approach, I have extended the noun *particle* into a verb, *particalization:* to break down into the smallest level. This act of particalization makes deconstruction and reintegration possible. Using the act of particalization as an interrogation technique, each of the materials of performance are established as being of the same importance as the artist. I believe that the process of particalization allows for helpful insights and a unique sense of physical integration with the materials that is not found in traditional performance training.

The Bridge forms a sort of double helix with the six materials by initiating discussions that reach beyond simply identifying the material structure of performance. These nine laboratories begin by tracing the origins of the Six Viewpoints and progress to a conclusion that draws a circle around the entire study.

The Bridge:

- discusses the process and results of microscopic examination
- examines the philosophies that continue to influence performer and audience interactions
- reviews the accumulated effects of the Viewpoints' interrogation of the materials

CHAPTER 7

News of a Difference Laboratory

Noticing Difference in Increasing Levels of Subtlety

THIS LABORATORY CONTAINS THE ORIGINAL SOURCE OF THE SIX VIEWPOINTS nonhierarchical process. In News of a Difference, performers, directors and choreographers are introduced to the details that surround them on a microscopic level. This laboratory suggests a way to communicate with the physical existence of theater as we might experience a landscape, as though performance were a part of nature. The concept of the philosophy and practice of News of a Difference expands awareness through a physical interrogation that collects minuscule, seemingly useless, details.

Each practice of the SSTEMS, found in the Six Viewpoints Practice Manual at the conclusion of this book, should be approached with the philosophy of News of a Difference (NOD).

CURRICULUM 1

INTRODUCTION

Students should understand that News of a Difference contains a guide for their practice. Repeated practices in Space, Shape, Time, Emotion, Movement and Story should be monitored to make sure that the materials are being interrogated on a highly detailed level. NOD advocates abstaining from making "theater" in order to support the subtle nuances of the SSTEMS languages. If the SSTEMS practices are completed too quickly, important Viewpoints foundational training will be missed. If the foundations instilled in the laboratory of News of a Difference are not mastered, nonhierarchical dialogue can easily slip back into traditional hierarchical creator/originator usage.

The Six Viewpoints' News of a Difference laboratory has more in common with oriental philosophy than with Western concepts of creativity. The concept of News of a Difference entered my creative practice with my journey into Transcendental Meditation. In the 1960s a wave of interest in Eastern meditation was just reaching U.S. soil. I remember Allen Ginsberg around 1965, recently returned from India, walking into the Fillmore West ballroom in San Francisco where all the big bands, The Grateful Dead, The Jefferson Airplane, etc., played. He was there to announce that he would lead a meditation at the end of the evening if anyone wanted to stay. I stayed. A few years later, in 1967, I learned that people were starting to do a technique known as TM. The purpose of this meditation was to refine your conscious awareness. It was said that it was not a religion, there was no dogma attached, you got your mantra and you were good to go.

About four years into meditating I began to apply this philosophy to my art process. I began to slow down and look more deeply into experiences and perceptions in dance classes and in choreography. In 1969 I discovered SoHo and moved there to work among a group of people who were engaged as artists in subtle deconstruction. I see these events as a wave of discovery in many iterations: a fascination with paying attention to details, contemplation as a viable end, intention as product, as art itself.

News of a Difference is an old TM term meaning noticing difference on finer and finer levels of the structure you are investigating. For me, this process manifested itself in a conceptual/philosophical way and unveiled a new, nonhierarchical approach to creating theater and dance.

This discovery of nonhierarchical structure led to transforming both the artists' and the audiences' roles into being dual observers/participants. In this definition the performers and audience are immersed in a purposefully structured environment which generates a particular perceptual stimulus. "Reading" the art becomes about one's own perceptions being challenged to evolve. There is a nonhierarchical presentation of the materials (the SSTEMS), challenging the artist and audience to read what is traditionally almost invisible.

> "American landscape painting in the nineteenth century . . . reveals a struggle with light and space that eventually set it apart from a contemporary European tradition of pastoral landscapes framed by trees, the world viewed from a carriage window. American painters meant to locate an actual spiritual presence in the North American landscape... The atmosphere of these paintings is silent and contemplative. They suggest a private rather than a public encounter with the land. Several critics . . . have described as well a peculiar "loss of ego" in the paintings. The artist disappears. The authority of the work lies, instead with the land. And the light in them is like a creature, a living, integral part of the scene. The landscape is numinous, imposing, real . . . "
>
> BARRY LOPEZ, *Arctic Dreams*

Perhaps this evolution toward "loss of ego" has been slowly overtaking American artists since we first landed on this continent. Certainly Montana seems to have been the grounding influence in my fascination with TM and minimalism.

News of a Difference requires a particular type of technical preparation. The performers' physical, mental, emotional, vocal, and visual training must be geared

CURRICULUM 2

news of a difference

News of a Difference is represented in the physical movement training methods I recommend. The physical training I teach is designed to cul- tivate attention to the finest level of perception and dialogue with the body. Performers should learn to communicate with great detail and practicality on a skeletal and muscular level—the muscle in the back of the knee, proximal extension, the function of the spine—training awareness from the tail bone to the cranium. Bring the pubic bone into relationship with the ileum. I categorize this type of training as "pre-movement" or foundational training. As performers acquire this degree of attention to their bodies, they become able to automatically develop a focus that contains a "News of a Difference" level of attention.

toward contemplation and awareness. In NOD, individuals must be given the chance to rely upon their own interior senses with little or no outside command or externally generated enthusiasm. To engage in this practice, you must take several actions:

Isolate and then focus on a subject: open your perceptions to every detail of it without a filter.

Give yourself permission to spend as much time as the subject demands of you; return to the subject again and again; allow what you see to change.

I made this level of attention manifest in the solo *Small Dance*. Taking a normal choreography, I removed the Space from a dance and performed only the remaining shifts of weight. The philosophy in *Small Dance* was to bring a dance to the audience that exposes them to News of a Difference. This solo makes its impact when the audience realizes their ability to perceive movement on a microscopic level.

Another example of the use of News of a Difference as a microscopic tool was applied to a collaboration with theater director Joanne Akalaitis in Dressed like an Egg. Akalaitis wanted the actors to communicate onstage in code. In looking at the possibilities I finally choose to approach the problem through the view of audience's perceptions. I thought that the real issue would be manipulating the audiences' focus rather than inventing a complicated coded system between the performers. The atmosphere of a code needed to be established by playing between what is seen and unseen by the audience. I cannot recall now whether it was I or Joanne who requested that the curtain be lowered so the audience sees only the feet of the performers. This I hoped would make the audience start to try to deduce what was happening. Putting the audience in the mind of code breaking, I had the actors tapping their feet and walking in patterns on the floor. There never was a real code, just the atmosphere of one. Causing the audience to participate in NOD by refusing to fully disclose what was going on onstage seemed amazingly effective. In this iteration, minute details brought great tension to the opening scene.

CHAPTER 8

Deconstruction Laboratory

Investigating Theater by Separating the Components of Its Structure

DECONSTRUCTION INTRODUCES THE TENSION OF THE OTHER TO THE Six Viewpoints contemplative dialogue. Open to including every detail, from the screws in the stage found in Space practice to the ability of being seen in your own presence through Emotion practice, the performer now must differentiate in more complex systems of engagement.

CURRICULUM 3

DECONSTRUCTION

I like to get students working with a difficult contrast within the SSTEMS, such as Time and Movement. These materials both involve principals of kinetics and sensation but come from very different origins. Movement is derived from sensation. Time derives from impulse which is precognitive sensation. With these two materials in close proximity, a performer interrogates one and then the other using improvisational investigation. With practice the difference between the two should become clear and articulate.

CURRICULUM 4

DECONSTRUCTION CONTINUED

A second step in deconstruction returns to Space: I suggest rolling on the floor to remove assumed artistic ownership or pedestrian command. To tap into the intelligence of "pure" Space, try making up an arbitrary blocking or floor pattern. Take a piece of paper and make a continuous line drawing without lifting the pen. It shouldn't have any connection to a specific piece you are currently working on. You are simply drawing. Then give it to an actor or dancer as a direction for dealing with the space in their choreography or play.

Approaching deconstruction through setting up contrasts between any two of the SSTEMS—Shape and Time, Movement and Space, Movement and Space—without blurring the distinctions develops greater facility. The articulation is forced to be more precise and so of higher performance value.

The skills developed in the Deconstruction Laboratory are observation and analysis. To begin to acquire these skills the performer must be given things to analyze that are separate from their own creativity.

Deconstruction is a delicate and exacting process: one distracted breath or flighty misstep throws you off course and you will not find any real challenge. If you use Space only for placing movements or for blocking dictated by a script you will be distracted by construction necessities and miss the information that pure deconstruction, keeping the parts separate, has to offer in terms of more dimensionality in your performances. Without a good grasp of deconstruction you will know little about what you are working with. To work effectively with the SSTEMS you must learn to make deconstructive distinctions.

In the Deconstruction Laboratory the voices of the six materials become bright and chatty. When the STTEMS are located, there is so much to pay attention to, so much high-level communication going on. Your study of Space might result in that material leading the creative dialogue. The Space might speak:

"This window ledge is really comfortable, dramatic and quietly contemplative. Maybe you should just invent a character for the window that is not in the play, or place a dancer here for the whole performance."

I like the words *proper deconstruction* in the context of this upside-down world where the materials can speak to us. To get a clear picture of what I mean by *proper deconstruction*, let's take an easier subject, say a shirt, rather than the huge subject of theater. To take a shirt apart to see how it is made without destroying it, we require some extremely sharp cutting tool, such as a razor blade. A very precise tool, a very observant eye, a deeply thoughtful mind and patience, allows us to investigate how this shirt is made. The seams must be opened, just as the stage must be opened, and each part—the sleeve, the collar, the pockets, the back, the front, and the cuffs—must remain intact. When a shirt is taken apart in this manner, the information about how the shirt is made is fully available. The person doing the deconstructing is then in a position to make a calculated and significant contribution by improvising with the parts to discover a new design logic.

Many key artists of the 20th and 21st centuries work with deconstruction. Their work has turned contemporary art inside out.

The composer John Cage, who created work from the 1930s until the mid-1990s, opened up the field of music and influenced many generations of artists in other mediums by showing that listening can create music out of daily sounds or random notes.

Beginning in the 1970s, the dancer and choreographer Steve Paxton deconstructed traditional dance and discovered that all dance has an unexamined mandatory space inserted between dancers. He questioned this odd finding and discovered (or uncovered) Contact Improvisation. Now we have a totally new form of dance with a very new "aha" message for its audience. It exposes the amazing kinetic possibilities that come from two human beings sharing one point of balance. The audience is exposed to a constantly changing flow of forms.

Dancer/choreographer Trisha Brown (like Paxton, a founding member of the Judson Dance Theater) discovered a released system of motion that has expanded the movement possibilities of dancers around the world. Her investigations do not place the body into held shapes and positions, but instead employ kinetics and mixed shapes with momentum. Brown focuses on the pendulum action of the limbs as both form and a means of locomotion.

Since the 1960s, the productions of theater director Robert Wilson have investigated time and space and given us modern icons of life on an operatic scale. In an early production he slowed down the action of the performers until a simple diagonal crossing was imperceptible. By deconstructing time he introduced staging as an immense visual picture.

Richard Serra's sculptures allow the viewer to contemplate form through the medium of space. His huge, curved pressed-steel walls that slant out from their base or retreat from the eye are primarily and uniquely communicated by means of the space they occupy.

In contemporary science as well as in contemporary art the results of deconstruction have been powerful and profound. With a great precision of focus, on a level of News of a Difference, deconstruction was used to split the atom. In the era of deconstruction and microscopic focus, our scientists are now discovering gene manipulation. We are scrutinizing brain function. We are microscopically investigating the earth, weather patterns, animal migrations, pollution, the oceans, fish populations, insects, and plant growth. We are looking at life more closely than ever before; we've uncovered troves of knowledge that we don't yet even know how to use. Performance and art are beginning to function on this level as well, and with this new focus we have no idea what we might be able to accomplish.

CHAPTER 9

The Horizontal Laboratory

Nonhierarchical Composition

THE HORIZONTAL LABORATORY REQUIRES MICROSCOPIC FOCUS AND "gin-clear" deconstruction (a term taken from World War II pilots, who would say at times they were able to fly in gin-clear skies). The Viewpoints definition, theory and practice of the horizontal is derived from an embrace of nonhierarchical structure: nonhierarchical refers to any situation characterized by impartiality. Horizontal differs slightly, extending the term to refer to a working condition in which an infinite number of new hierarchies may be formed and dissolved. As a working condition, the Horizontal Laboratory fosters training in complex reasoning which then multiplies performative resources. In this laboratory, with no preferential point of view, information can be perused by experimental means. Any juxtaposition of the SSTEMS, outside scripts, objects, timings, sources, etc. can be rearranged to form temporary hierarchies.

All systems of reasoning—mathematics, medicine, philosophy, computer sciences, the arts, etc.—require training. The Six Viewpoints reasoning training begins in establishing an understanding of deconstruction. Immersing the performer in six discrete languages, the SSTEMS, achieves the first step in complex reasoning. The second step is to deconstruct and introduce nonhierarchy. The third step, horizontality, introduces a fully performative activity.

CURRICULUM 5

OPEN SSTEMS IMPROVISATION

This practice provides the first schooling in horizontal interaction for performers. In Open SSTEMS Improvisation all performers are free to use any and all SSTEMS as free languages between them. This practice begins to make an environment of individual development. There are no other rules. Every SSTEMS practice leads to this training ground. Weeks of interrogating each of the materials must precede any attempt at this practice. Open SSTEMS Improvisation is a chance to inhabit a performative dimension that is an equal mixture of choice and chance. In many ways this practice is like a giant artistic game of basketball.

The concept of the Horizontal came to me in the late eighties. I had been struggling to discover a physical, visual way to express the nonhierarchical world that deconstruction opens to performance. I decided to employ takeout cups from the Greek deli on the corner of Broadway and Waverley Street. I used them to represent each of the SSTEMS. They stack so beautifully into what I called solid state theater, all the SSTEMS joined in one action, rehearsal, play or choreography. Yet they could be separated into equal, nonprejudicial units.

Unfortunately it was never quite as smooth as I had wished. Inevitably I lost control when six were free in my hands. Ending up ignominiously scattered over the floor before I was able to complete the sentence " . . . you can build anything you want . . . ." Several years into this practice, as the cups scattered on to the floor once again, rather than rushing to explain further, I paused to honor the ridiculousness of the moment. In this tiny break an epiphany occurred. The cups were lying horizontally! The floor took on a philosophical importance, delivering a tangible condition to work in. In this horizontally supported position I could pick one up without disturbing the others. I could pick up two and begin to build an experimental structure free of the stack. I had a wildly experimental situation in front of me. The Viewpoints Horizontal Laboratory thus found articulation, circa 1990.

The Horizontal Laboratory facilitates a remarkably fluid environment for experimentation. These are the conditions existing in the laboratory:

The concept of the nonhierarchical avoids conflict and makes experimentation a stable, playful, and expanding experience, because hierarchy, necessarily present in any structure, is seen as temporary. Construction of hierarchies can come and go as rapidly as you need. In other words, the assumptions that accompany hierarchical thinking (the pressure to be right, the pressure to be original, the assumption that it is your job to adopt a chosen structure as soon as possible) is set aside. The Horizontal Laboratory frees you of this pressure. When you walk into the Performing Garage, the Wooster Group's physical theater at 72 Wooster Street in New York, you are standing in a fully operative nonhierarchical plant. You know immediately that you will never know what is going on until you see opening night. What stabilizes this type of exploration is the presence of a clear philosophical overview.

I often refer to processes in the Horizontal Laboratory as rerouting information or connecting new circuits. In this laboratory it's as though each of the SSTEMS contains electrical circuitry that can be commandeered into almost infinite patterns. Each new connection illuminates a new awareness, a new way to drive the narrative, a new way to approach a character, a new way of approaching movement, a new way of choreographing in space.

This property of "switching on a light," or arcing, in the Horizontal Laboratory only occurs when one has been trained to be in a state of mind that is open to new perspectives and new levels of awareness. This training in the Viewpoints comes through being able to work in the laboratories of News of a Difference and Deconstruction—in other words, to particalize. This is why these laboratories are so important to the Viewpoints perspective. They prepare the artist to put aside any determined effort to produce a product, and instead to create space for contemplation. There must be the willingness and technical preparedness to throw everything out, work blind for days or months or years, make and tear down

CURRICULUM 6

THE FIFTH STORY

Another much more advanced practice not only interrogates Story/ Logic but is also an excellent example of nonhierarchical properties of the Horizontal. Gathering into groups of four performers, bring a array of diverse reading material: poetry, sociology, political analysis, biology, novels and essays. The group will be constructing a fifth story as they work in the horizontal conditions of non-compatible books. (Books with titles containing surnames, such as history texts or biographies, do not work well in the practice. If, during the course of this practice, a reader finds they have no chance to contribute to the reading then they should choose another book.)

The rules are:

1. Choose to start at any place in the book that appeals to you. Once you have chosen the starting point, you must deliver every word, consecutively, as written. You must not skip text to please your own creative taste.

2. No reader is allowed to speak a whole sentence. The others must complete the story by continuing the sentence, adding to the plot that is emerging.

3. The words each reader contributes must make logical sense. This is not an abstract practice.

4. In order to create the logic of the Fifth Story, the words must be read with timing and emotional emphasis even if the readers do not know where they are going.

hierarchical structures and finally to recognize when you have found something.

In the process of this practice, the readers are actively engaged in simultaneous horizontal listening and action. As they work, a skill develops enabling them to become a highly trained observer/participant by challenging their mental agility and technical conceptual recognition.

In the Fifth Story we experience the strange property of the Horizontal Laboratory: the idea that if we control information too early, it has much less dynamic energy, and fewer lessons to impart. The stories that emerge from a successful session of the Fifth Story contain thoughts no one has ever heard before. They are creations of the observer/participant functioning in a horizontal encounter, and carry within their particalized structure potential ways of expressing and connecting that cross the boundaries of our hierarchical fixed processes.

Here is a sample sentence taken from a Fifth Story process:

> "Not another word was printed, it was accidental, but the reason it was
> in the room, in Vienna, it was so useful, it would age with a rotting floor."

These are the books we used: *Nerds 2.0.1: A Brief History of the Internet* by Stephen Segaller; *Dictionary of the Khazars: A Lexicon Novel* by Milorad Pavić; *The London Embassy* by Paul Theroux; *The Lost City* by John Gunther.

Making performance from the nonhierarchical Horizontal Laboratory can be like having IKEA deliver a piece of furniture to your house. The pieces are disassembled, just as theater is when it arrives in the Horizontal. Of course directions about how to make theater and dance surround us in traditional productions, just as the IKEA product arrives with instructions. But the challenge of the Horizontal is akin to your IKEA purchase arriving without those pictogram instructions.

Imagine that, just as with your IKEA order, the parts of theater and dance are strewn about on the floor, the Horizontal. In the Six Viewpoints we have the six materials which have subsets of pieces.

Space contains blocking, placement of furniture, placement of the walls, doors and windows, angle of gaze, distance of projection, and spatial alignment of the actors to the proscenium, to the audience, and to each other, etc.

Shape contains geometry, costumes, gestures, and the shape of the actors' bodies and of all the objects onstage.

Time contains duration, rhythm, punctuation, pattern, impulse, repetition, legato, pizzicato, lyrical, rhythm, and a myriad of unnamed qualities of movement.

Emotion contains presence, anger, laughter, pensiveness, empathy, alienation, romance, pity, fear, anticipation, etc.

Movement contains falling, walking, running, blood pumping, breath, suspension, contraction, impact, etc.

Story contains logic, order and progression of information, memory, projection, conclusions, allusions, truth, lies, associations, influences, power, weakness, reification, un-reification, construction, and deconstruction, etc.

The Horizontal affords the luxury of studying each of these subjects from any entrance into structure. To demonstrate the vastness of this lab, let's return to your Ikea purchase. Imagine that four articles arrived from IKEA and that none of them were labeled or separated out in anyway. Here you are with all these screws and hinges and doors and crossbars. Now suppose that you had no idea what it was that you had ordered. No picture of the chair, the bed, the shelves. No universal instructions. You might very well end up with a sixteen-foot couch with three shelves underneath and doors that form part of the back of the couch that slide up and hold a coffee maker or computer, or extra pillows for a change of color scheme. Perhaps the couch gives rise to a whole concept called the chameleon home. This possibility is your playground in the Horizontal.

A fascinating possibility came about in SoHo: that we can entertain ideas that are too big for us to see or experience in one sitting. This idea I believe belongs to the

CURRICULUM 7

POOL ON AN EGG-SHAPED TABLE

The "pool" table is the shape of an egg cut in half the long way and hollowed out till the shell is all that remains. The table, rather than being flat, is an egg-shaped bowl. Imagine playing pool on this table. Because of its odd and complex shape, it would be impossible to predict the path of a shot as the ball careens wildly inside this bowl. The outcome of your or anyone's actions is beyond control yet you proceed to play the game.

The game: Each performer adopts their own individual focus, metaphorically turning their back on the other performers. Each must generate exclusive material, motivations, timing, shapes, space, kinetics, logic and presence. Participants may not use any material other than their own. Ensemble members may not relate to the other performers in time, gesture, logic, space, kinetics or in any other manner. Each performer has their own material, which is unique and unrelated to the material of any other performers. All the participants perform their improvisation simultaneously, maintaining the absolute autonomy of their material.

Horizontal Laboratory. Choreographer Trisha Brown created a spatial pattern in "Glacial Decoy" that was too big for the stage. In the process of performing beautifully elaborate traveling steps the dancers would appear and disappear on a giant circle that extended off stage. The dance has a wonderful expansive effect on me when I have the privilege to see it.

An advanced level of the Horizontal Laboratory can be employed after work in Open SSTEMS Improvisation: the following practice actually removes almost all dialogue with the materials as partners. In it the element of nonhierarchy is foremost while the performer is placed in an observer/participant roll with the emphasis on observation.

Performers in the laboratory are united by the thinnest connection. They are required to occasionally glance over their shoulders to check out what is going on in the room. The tension between their independence and this awareness of the other is what makes this practice valuable as an extreme training process for the Horizontal. No one is being allowed to make a connection. They can only observe the connections as they flow along in the process. If cooperation should accidentally occur it must not be allowed to steer the performers into a lengthy collaboration. If they come together by accident they should work together only so long as the internal logic of each performer's separate project compels them do so.

Imagine performance being a long string of pearls and that the string breaks. The pearls scatter and bounce everywhere, even over all boundaries of our imaginations and expectations of cause and effect.

CHAPTER 10

Postmoderism Laboratory

The Philosophical Foundation

ENTERING THE POSTMODERNISM LABORATORY, WE ARE NOW LOCATED at the heart of the Six Viewpoints. The preceding laboratories are, to me, an approach to making art that formulates a postmodern practice. The heart of Postmodernism rests in the microscopic activity of differentiation, which is found in the laboratories of News of a Difference, Deconstruction and the Horizontal. These laboratories are reflected most starkly in the nonhierarchical approach that the Viewpoints take to the materials of the SSTEMS in both practice and concept. It is not imperative that you adopt Postmodernism after reading this book or studying the Viewpoints. As with all artistic processes, the artist will take what they want and what has significance to them.

Many regard Postmodernism to be dead. In my opinion they are referring to a mistaken idea of Postmodernism that rests on bad deconstruction and collage. I agree that this version of Postmodernism has passed. It is deserted because there was no depth to the "innovation" to begin with. The type of Postmodernism I present in this laboratory is very different and in my opinion is hugely consequential for the art of this century, and is in its infancy.

Universities require art students to study the history and philosophies of their discipline whether it is law, mathematics, language or the arts. This knowledge is regarded as imperative in order to be well prepared, well educated. This laboratory adopts that perspective by presenting a practical and practicable connection to the philosophy of Postmodernism. Since each practice found in the Six Viewpoints Practice Manual and the first three laboratories forms a step-by-step foundation to Postmodernism, you find this philosophy in the center of the Bridge. In this connection Postmodernism is the core double helix that exists in the relationship between the Bridge and the SSTEMS. The nonhierarchical principles found in Deconstruction and the Horizontal are key components of Postmodernism, and the Six Viewpoints are deeply entwined with this philosophy. To study the SSTEMS is to study Postmodernism in a practical medium.

The Bridge's Postmodernism Laboratory was not sourced from academic influence. It evolved as the art of SoHo evolved and as the structure of the Viewpoints took shape from within. This often poorly understood, at times ponderous and even preposterously flexible, ill-defined and unusual philosophy arises in the middle of the Bridge as anatural extension of News of a Difference, Deconstruction and the Horizontal. I've put such a controversial and some think passé philosophy into the middle of the Bridge because understanding the relationship between the Six Viewpoints and Postmodernism is an important part of being well educated as a Six Viewpoints-influenced artist. The Postmodernism Laboratory helps underscore the importance of the artist as the dual observer/participant. This laboratory also introduces dancers and actors to the principal artists of the seventies and eighties, the era when a new nonhierarchical mindset took root. This laboratory makes it possible to understand the reasons for the development of these innovations, and to employ the concepts properly.

The shift to Postmodernism is easily identified by examining the dramatic changes that took place in dance in the late sixties, seventies and eighties.

Altering the process of making dance, thehierarchical relationshiptoa choreographer as sole creator was replaced by improvisation and group collaboration.

Traditional dance techniques were stripped away, opening the door to a vast number of new, investigative techniques based on new resources: anatomy; brain development; touch; memory, etc. The acceptance of everyday physical motion and the "elegant pedestrian," as Barbara Dilley refers to it, was introduced to performance.

The individual dancer came to be regarded as an artist, not just a performer.

With all these changes choreography also stepped into a freer more choreographer-specific creative process. The swinging of the arms and legs became a kinetic signature in the work of Trisha Brown; walking, running skipping became the foundation of the immensely minimalistic and mathematically complex work of choreographer Lucinda Childs; and balancing one body against another opened a portal into a universe of movement when dancer Steve Paxton developed Contact Improvisation.

Dance, along with all the other disciplines, moved away from statements and products towards nonhierarchical concern with the function of moving and processes of perception. A perfect and easily seen example of this is the sudden adoption of loose, soft flowing dance wear. Essentially, the whole concept of costumes that expose the body vanished at the start of this period, as sweat pants, and later pedestrian clothing, took over. In this choice of costume and practice wear, postmodern dance was making a statement that movement should be unrestricted. Many regard Postmodernism as a heady esoteric and difficult philosophy. But in its manifestation in the dance of the seventies it was a grounded and inclusive study that integrated microscopic examination with humanist values.

Philosophy is to me something that you are engaged in every day. It can be found in the style of your clothing, the structure of your relationships and the way you define the purpose and path of your life. It is an important way to articulate social trends. The manifestation of philosophy through art is inextricably linked with social and cultural developments. A painting, a music score, a dance can reflect our thoughts in ways that no other activity can match.

I caution my students about who they are dealing with by pronouncing in my classes that I am a card-carrying Postmodernist. In this way they can make up their own minds about my opinions and know the background of my approach. I believe it serves the artist well to understand the philosophy they are referencing, whether it is their own or that of an era, or a combination of philosophies.

The biggest challenge in establishing this laboratory is to clearly define Postmodernism. I believe that few have a clear concept of the structure of this philosophy. Modernism, with its unifying belief in hierarchy, was easier to join. Modernists were looking for the truth, the answer, and they were sure that these were possible to find.

Although I felt I understood Postmodernism, the comprehension of this philosophy had only been accomplished through embracing the artistic products of my generation. Any more intellectual abstract articulation was frustratingly out of reach.

My first major confusion surrounding Postmodernism in the abstract was that I had no way of articulating nonhierarchical situations. I could witness nonhierarchical manifestation in the improvisation, choreography, music and visual arts that surrounded me. The processes of News of a Difference, Deconstruction and the Horizontal would have to come first as I worked to analyze what was happening inside the Viewpoints themselves: the minimalistic, super-detailed focus, the separation of elements, the nonhierarchical composition.

In the art world I entered in 1970, Modernist values created a tension and confrontation that made it difficult to analyze such things as improvisational dance, Contact Improvisation, non-scripted theater, and Happenings. In short, the art of that time was on a skirmish line as judged by Modernist values. Downtown artists were under attack as lacking technique, time-honored ego-centered creative values or final products that held together and could be sold on the market. Today those powerful suspicions and judgments about nonhierarchical structure have vanished and the new values—postmodern values—have been digested, so much so that even corporate capitalists look for ways to profit off this philosophy. The detailed, individualized and horizontal approach to structure is finding thousands of new products for us to consume on a monthly basis, such as open-source software and millions of free apps.

Modernism's belief in discovering universal truths has been much discussed. Many good things came out of Modernism, but also a great deal of prejudice and judgmental attitudes. Postmodernists come from a quite different orientation, with their minute differentiation, nonprejudicial examination for examination's sake, and democratization of all data. Postmodernism, by adopting a pluralistic Both/ And approach, challenges the very basis of Modernism.

The Six Viewpoints, originating from within a Postmodernist stance, turn away from the Modernist ideal of the artist as sole creator/originator and reject the idea of a single universal truth.

After casting about for many years knowing Postmodernism by example but unable to articulate its structure, I came across an article in 1989, in the Royal Danish University library in Copenhagen, that rescued me. The paper, by professors Nicholas Burbules and Susan Rice, was on postmodern education.

Their amazingly clear work gave me a structure that allowed me to communicate my own physical and artistic experiences of Postmodernism. Until I read their work, I could not define Postmodernism—even though I was sure that my work was postmodern. This certainty was based on the fact that I knew it was not modern or classical. I adopted the term postmodern from a dance review by Sally Banes written in the 1970s. I knew instantly that it also applied to my work. I was a Postmodernist! Like most people in that time I used the term but could only give a definition by using examples of art that I felt represented its principles. If the person I was talking to did not know any of the artists I mentioned, I was helpless. It was profoundly embarrassing that I could not define the philosophy I had adopted years earlier.

In their work at that time, Burbules and Rice created a clear definition of Postmodernism by contrasting it with the two preceding major philosophies, Classicism and Modernism. Each of these philosophies has a specific line of investigation and perspective.

While these three philosophies differ dramatically in their goals and means of inquiry, and although the transition to Postmodernism had a great deal of conflict,

I believe that their differences do not represent inherent negation, competition or conflict.

Classicism

I like to define Classicism by standing with my arms reaching skyward along with my gaze. This philosophy is based on a belief that there is a divine order and purity to nature. Classical investigation focused on the order of the planets, gravity in relationship to physical materials such as weight and flow of water, structures such as arches, and the structure of the body in relationship to these great principles. This study was founded in a belief that there is a hierarchy to this information. Nature is a manifestation of divine perfection, and following that logic, only the very noblest of people—kings, clergy, and high scholars—have the blessings of divine order that allow them access to this information.

Our entire civilization is based on classical discoveries. We live in buildings of many stories, understand that the sun is at the center of our universe, that our planet is round, and that we are one of many planets that circle the sun. We could not function without this information; it is the foundation of all that we empirically know. We have classical dance, discovered and founded on the anatomical principles of the body and the spirals, rotations, and functions of weight placement. This is the foundation of all Western dance. Classical art focused on depicting the sublime, the lofty, grand, or exalted in thought, expression, or manner.

Modernism

In my non-conflicted version of the evolution of these philosophies, Modernism evolved out of the principals of Classicism. As Classicism began to wane, we asked: if nature is perfect and therefore an example of divine order, then is not mankind also a part of God's creation and worthy of investigation? Based on this questioning, which turned into a revelatory and then a revolutionary vision (the Reformation), Modernism sprang into being led by, among others, Martin Luther. A simple question turned everything around.

I like to depict Modernism by reaching forward, holding my arms straight out from my chest, horizontally. I gesture, reaching toward another human being, then put my hand to my chest and then back to the person. Modernism was the result of a process that took Classicism's view and extended it to common humankind. Being a part of nature, man must also be capable of perfection. Modern ideology began to look into the affairs of man. The hierarchy of Classicism drooped to eye level, and a new investigation, "the revolution," began. This philosophy looked into the nature of our minds, our emotions, and our bodies. Western man found that human beings were capable of learning. The printing press was invented, schools for everyone were established, new systems of government were instituted believing that all people are able to determine their own destiny. Hospitals were founded to take care of the population. Mass production evolved to give all peoples the right to clothing, household goods and food. Democracy was invented, along with Socialism and Communism—ways for people to determine the structure they would live and cooperate under. Freud began to investigate what went on inside the mind. New ideas of how people could produce food were introduced, as were ideas of exporting these systems to the rest of the world. Common people were now seen as capable of organizing themselves, establishing disciplines and investigating our inner truths. The art of Modernism focuses on what motivates people, influencing their relationships and their mental processes.

Postmodernism

I depict Postmodernism by lying on the floor in the position of the prone Buddha. Modernism studied the human condition, and Postmodernism took this concern one step further. With its insistence on nonhierarchy, Postmodernism took into account every detail of the individual rather than grouping people into categories and classes. Minorities of all persuasions began to be viewed as independent and unique human beings. On the level of the planet, all details of the natural environment began to be respected in their own right as critical parts of an ecosystem. Likewise, the Viewpoints reflect this quest by seeking to find and release as equal players each of the basic structural materials of theater.

This investigation began a revelation and a revolution as we stopped seeking empirical all-inclusive knowledge systems and instead chose to particalize subjects in order to get a better understanding of what things are made of and how they function. Particle investigation brought about the unavoidable collapse of hierarchy; the idea that one thing is better or more important than the other was no longer a viable stance to take. In fact, it obstructed research and growth. In the Viewpoints all the materials are held to be equal, and with this stance an amazing variety of staging, subject matter, and acting and dancing possibilities have opened up. Performance can say and do more now. This is simply not a Modernist stance.

To demonstrate particle philosophy, I make my point by approaching a woman in my classroom and asking if it would be all right to take her away from the group for a moment. Standing with her in front of the class, I point out that this woman possesses characteristics that make her totally unique. In the modern era this woman would be seen as a member of a subcategory called woman, housewife, mother, wife, or simply married or not married. Previously, looking beyond these "facts" did not occur to people because it did not serve the function of Modernism with its quest for unifying and universal principles. Now, however, she is seen, along with all peoples on earth, as a distinct, powerful, individual entity. To me this is a sweeping and almost silent change that has occurred and is still occurring as the process of individuation moves deeper into our lives and into the structure of society.

Surveying this complexity, one may wonder how I dare insert a dialogue on the structure of the Six Viewpoints into a Postmodernism Laboratory. I have a number of justifications:

First, I think the Viewpoints make Postmodernism easy to understand and accessible through exposure of its principles.

Secondly, I believe that artists who are aware of their philosophical context engage in a living dialogue with their time.

Thirdly, I believe that art with a clear philosophical background is more likely to remain of value for many generations as a dialogue with deep, insightful information.

And lastly, art and artists aware of philosophy help to make it accessible to society and strengthen that philosophy's principles through practice.

Contrary to what many think, I believe we are only at the beginning of the era of Postmodernism and we desperately need to learn to drive our postmodern philosophical vehicle. I believe that if we can learn to navigate its principles, investigating and applying nonhierarchical structure, inclusive of Both/And interrogations and maintaining a deep connection to nature, we will find ourselves living in a world that is based on expanded equality, empathic and life-sustaining beyond any Modernist's dreams.

If we can't learn to operate this philosophy, we will not be in touch with our destiny nor that of our planet. The art of the seventies successfully established nonhierarchical, Both/And principles, and if better understood, those valuable perceptual processes can be developed and furthered by many generations to come. In this way, this laboratory and the entire Six Viewpoints structure is devoted to better comprehension and navigation of nonhierarchical structures. The practices in this book can and have helped people perceive and engage the world from a different point of view. The beauty of this Both/And philosophy is that there is no need to destroy what has been given to us by our Classical and Modern eras. Those perspectives simply get folded into this era of Postmodernism.

There are many aspects of this postmodern vehicle that are intensely unfamiliar and just downright confusing to us. Its metaphoric steering wheel affords navigational ability that is still beyond many people's comprehension. Various models can move sideways, change directions, switching at any moment what is front and what is back. We live with this reality already. We call about our bank account and unwittingly find that we are talking to someone in India; we bounce communication off a round object orbiting in space. We can turn a light on in our house when we are thousands of miles away and create circles of friends that cover many countries and continents. This is the nonhierarchical, particalized, rapid-fire creativity of the incidental, and our children are more than ready for it.

In the Six Viewpoints there is no right way; there is an ever-expanding multitude of ways. Postmodernism took hierarchy and made it contingent on point of view. Shall we view theater from the aspect of Space or Time, or Emotion, or Movement, etc? In this new philosophy, structures (or at least our view of them) are understood to be in a state of flux. In Postmodernism, disagreement is viewed with interest, as an opportunity to learn, rather than as a threat to stability. In this new philosophy, hierarchies are gained by a process of finding points of relatedness in divergent details. It is all about details and interaction, rather than grand fixed plans. This is expressed in the Viewpoints in the fact that the training relies on improvisational structures as its primary method. The individual is trained to act as an independent responsive agent at all times.

The Viewpoints want independent actors who know how to swim within the six materials. When these actors are conscious of what surrounds them, they are capable of being in the moment and fully owning the work they produce onstage as responsible and independent individuals. In my opinion this is one of the greatest outcomes of Postmodernism.

I take the view that each of these philosophies, Classicism, Modernism and Postmodernism, are simply focuses that expose information in different ways in order to illuminate our surroundings, core challenges, and possible futures. Each philosophy evolved out of necessity and has specific outcomes. Furthermore I think that each approach has always existed. What makes one philosophy more prevalent in a particular era is the need of its perspective at that point in our evolution.

Mistaken Postmodernism

In the process of defining my ideas on the structure of Postmodernism, it is important to point out that there is a deep confusion between Postmodernism and what Rice and Burbles called Anti-Modernism. They postulate that Anti-Modernism believes that we are so individual that we can not share or understand each other's meaning, ideas or feelings. In their opinion, this Anti-Modernism is similar to the Existentialist movement in the Modern era. I found this distinction very helpful since there seemed to be many pieces of supposed postmodern literature that seemed to be outside my understanding of the philosophy. Whether you agree or disagree I think it is useful to have to think about this difference. Postmodernism is based in deconstruction and nonhierarchy; Anti-Modernism is based in a collage-like process. The collage seemingly follows a deconstructionist approach to separating elements in preparation for reassembling them in a new form. As I wrote in chapter 8, Deconstruction, to be of any research value the work has to be very disciplined and precise. Collage, although it may, on the surface, look like a deconstruction, is actually executed as an arbitrary series of unrelated actions.

This confusion leads to what I call Kitsch Postmodern Art, because it represents a misunderstanding of the process and purpose of deconstruction, and the possibilities and real use of horizontal composition. Although the art coming from a collage-like process can be powerful, beautiful and meaningful, it is important to know the difference. Collage deconstructions are bits and pieces from many sources placed together. Remember the carefully deconstructed shirt, razor blade, and seams? Kitsch Postmodernists might "deconstruct" the shirt by cutting the sleeve at the bicep or the body of the shirt down a diagonal, rendering the shirt unusable as either a future pattern for variations or a reusable item that could be reconstructed back into a whole. In Kitsch Postmodernism, the horizontal is mostly a copied attitude of style and for the most part is not useful as a process for evoking more subtle meaning.

CHAPTER 11

Reification Laboratory

A Reflection on Creativity, Communication, and Language

THIS LABORATORY INTERROGATES THE EXISTENCE OF ART. AS ARTISTS we occupy a special place in the cycles of progress. The act of reification is our real medium no matter what branch of art we have chosen. The Reification Laboratory represents the formulation of languages to communicate new ideas.

Just as I had articulated the Horizontal Laboratory with fallen paper cups, I simplified the concept of reification by drawing a big circle on a piece of paper. Contained in the center of the circle is all that we know as human beings. Outside the circle is all that we don't know. Artists and scientists must find their own process to enable them to escape the circle, reach into the unknown, discover something new, and then finally manage to bring the discovery back intact and communicate it to others. I had been functioning in this world as both artist and phenomenologist for a very long time. I felt, and still do feel, that without any college degrees or certificates, I had become a truly educated person.

I realized that the artist and the phenomenologist were united and that both were reifiers. Within every generation of artists, those who understand the core purpose of reification will make more effective and affecting art.

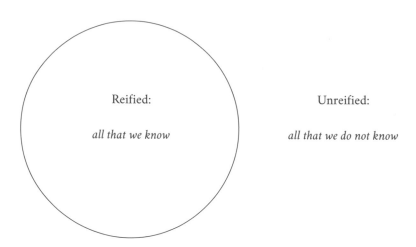

Reified:

all that we know

Unreified:

all that we do not know

In this practice students risk seeing if their findings can make viable performance, and get to see their friends make interesting art outside the normal framework. Because reification requires a witness, the group interaction and feedback is important.

I first encountered the concept underlying reification in 1968. I was in Estes Park, Colorado attending a teacher training course in Transcendental Meditation. Instead of leaving as a teacher, I left with a clear sense of the responsibility I was taking on in choosing to be an artist. It was soon after this experience that I began a new life in New York City as a member of the Natural History of the American Dancer. For the rest of my life I have studied, and have discovered practices and processes that allow me to bring ideas to life for others.

I was there with about 300 people who were all training to become teachers of Transcendental Meditation. Our lives revolved around "rounding" (20 minutes of meditation combined with a brief set of yoga postures). In the evening we listened to lectures by Maharishi. Maharishi was focused on investigating the connection of the sciences to TM.

There were about 30 artists at this course, and we asked to have a private meeting Maharishi. We gathered in the auditorium one afternoon. In his charming English he opened the meeting by saying: "So, you have some question for me?" One person immediately raised their hand, "Maharishi, can you help me? I do not know if I am

CURRICULUM 8

GRAZING

"Grazing" begins with a small team of students who are sent out of the classroom to choose a piece of the urban environment nearby. They are instructed to study this limited area for 20 minutes. Their attention must be restricted to the smallest details: shadows, vibration of sounds, movement of hinges in doors, etc. At the end of that time, spent in total silence, they are instructed to bring back the information and perform their findings.

Could this be theater? The participants experience reifying on an unusual scale that is as communicative, performable and readable as lines in Shakespeare. They have brought some new performance into the studio.

an artist or not." Maharishi looked out at us and said, "Are there others with this question?" About seven people raised their hands. Then in a very sweet voice he said, "If you have this question, you should leave the room." We were all stunned, and in the silence they quietly left.

He explained: "The rest of you also do not need to be here. Artists have their own personal meditations. If you choose to be here at this course that is fine, but it is not absolutely necessary for you." He lifted both his hands and indicated his right hand. "This is the sannyasi, the monk. They forswear the householder life and retreat into a cave to seek enlightenment." Then he moved his gaze to his left hand and said: "This is the artist. They dive into life, swim in it, play and try to experience everything they can. The artist and the monk share the same goals in terms of evolutionary activities. They are both seeking enlightenment but their practices are very different. The artist experiences and goes through the very center of life. When he or she is ready they choose a medium to work in, and their job is to instill that medium with as much consciousness as they can, and then to communicate this to their audiences. When their 'meditation' is done they present their work to raise the consciousness of the people. The more consciousness infused in the work, the longer it will remain important and interesting to the audience. Art with the highest levels of consciousness becomes what we know as classic."

Unfortunately, as influencing as this TM message was, my education was incomplete. I understood the mission of the artist but had no vocabulary with which to express this concept in writing or in a larger frame other than my own work. Years later, in 1986, having finished a great deal of work with the SSTEMS practices, I began my first attempts to write the Six Viewpoints down. After working for more that a year I realized that I was missing a concrete way to talk about this function of discovery and articulation that Maharishi described.

The frustration was overwhelming and caused me to begin to doubt myself and the entire theory. What was I doing? What were the Viewpoints? Was it all just hot air? It took many painful years before I finally ran into the information I lacked. When I made the discovery it turned out to be an explicit picture that succinctly explained what I had learned in that lecture long ago in Estes Park.

In the midst of my inner war with writing down the Viewpoints, I happened to be teaching at the School for New Dance Development in Amsterdam, in 1987. I attended a workshop, "The Relationship of Space to Human Thinking," organized by the artist Christina Svane, and led by a relatively obscure American high school teacher, thinker and writer, Robert Schwartz. I was amazed when he introduced the concept of reification. Without the unwitting intervention of Robert and Christie, this book would never have been written.

It turned out that there were two parts of me and they did not talk to each other very often and had no idea how they were related. One had searched for and found the Six Viewpoints. The other had a much looser way of functioning. She would just enter her studio and ask the question, what is on my mind, where should we start? This second person, the artist, was confused by the first person, the phenomenologist.

The phenomenologist understood that at some point she would be obliged to record

CURRICULUM 9

REIFICATION

The Viewpoint performer should know this term. As a student studies the SSTEMS, they carry the concept of Reification within each practice. I am reifying Space by being able to witness it as I stand in Space. I am reifying Shape by being able to perceive Shape in my body. I am reifying Time by feeling it course through my nervous system. I am reifying Emotion by being present in the moment and allowing myself to be witnessed. I am reifying Movement by acknowledging that it is a living force that I respond to. I am reifying Story by acknowledging that Logic is indispensable to life.

As a teaching practice, I focus on the process of Reification that my students are going through. I comment on who can see her arm now! That he is fully functional in Space. That this group is very gifted in Time, etc. That this student is not experiencing Space. I try to make it clear that they are not learning fixed information; they are processing information and experiencing the chemistry of Reification.

this theory and practice, since finding this language was an integral part of the mission. The artist quailed at the prospect of fixed words on a page. She had a consuming fear that they might, in some unknown way, damage the creative process.

This gap of understanding between the artist and the phenomenologist kept inhibiting me in my attempt to write. I developed a tiny voice in the back of my mind that kept saying, "Don't write this down, it might hurt people, all these labels!" In addition to hurting someone I thought, "you might expose a terrible ignorance that is hidden somewhere in the Six Viewpoints and end up looking like an idiot." That first fear of damaging artists proved to be untrue but was impossible to dismiss until I found

Reification. The second fear of being exposed as ignorant proved to be absolutely true. There was a lack of understanding of my own relationship to the Viewpoints. The concept of Reification would solve that problem as well.

I took the fated workshop in Amsterdam. I absolutely had to go because it was related to Space, even though I resist learning new things (they keep changing my universe). The first part is a blur. At midpoints in the workshop we were being introduced to the concept of reification, and as an exercise were asked to spend a weekend without our concept of Space. We were told that Space was just a label and not the total definition of what exists as space. Robert pointed the way for us by stating that we think of space as empty but that this concept is absolutely false.

That weekend I alternated between euphoria and complete terror. In the end we all returned to class with a very good idea of what Robert was referring to when he instructed us in the principles of reification. As that class on Monday unfolded, my understanding of art, thinking, the Viewpoints, dancing, reading, walking into the unknown all began to appear as one whole cloth. It felt like a miracle.

With the introduction of the concept of Reification I was rescued from a great ignorance and given a much larger picture of my profession, how it functioned, and how everything fit together from the beginning of time. We label (reify) our findings, creating a vocabulary with which to communicate to others what we have experienced, and we keep our universes stable and connected through these agreed upon definitions. These languages contain our history and our future as we connect and use the languages we discover.

Many people—both artist and non-artist—do not like the idea of having to face this constant challenge. Reifying is not a safe, secure activity; it requires the willingness to take a risk and live in a constantly changing world. You never know when something will shift, like the L subway line going out of service at 8:30 Monday morning. Think of it: thousands of people must re-reify the way they are going to get to work. They are forced to be creative and problem solve. However, if we take the leap into the unknown and make it back with something new, we become pioneers!

CHAPTER 12

The Piano Laboratory

The Interface Between Artist and Audience

THE PIANO LABORATORY COMPLETES THE SIX VIEWPOINTS PERSPECTIVE by taking up a philosophical and practical interrogation of the audience. Following the macroscopic laboratories of Postmodernism and Reification, the Piano Laboratory suddenly flips the SSTEMS from their position in the interrogation of the stage and performance to an interrogation of the audience.

In this interrogation the audience is seen as containing the SSTEMS, and can be regarded by the artist as an instrument much like a piano, containing keys upon which the artist plays the performance. The following practice can be used at virtually any time in the class.

CURRICULUM 10

PRESENCE PRACTICE

This curriculum may be the first thing you introduce, even before the SSTEMS, or it may be the last. I find that I usually like to win the confidence of the students before introducing this practice, but it can also be a fascinating way to begin. It all depends how quickly you can establish trust in the classroom. Whenever you choose to bring in this practice, it will profoundly change the students' perspective on performing. The Piano Laboratory makes use of the Presence Practice from the SSTEMS. It allows performers to examine the sensitivity of the audience by acknowledging their presence as witnesses.

The performer sits in a chair in front of the class. They practice allowing the audience to see them and at times look directly in their eyes. The performer practices thinking, breathing and feeling in the presence of the audience, and practice not blocking the audience's presence and ability to witness them. With this practice the performer can make the leap to the Piano: if the audience can see them think, feel and breath they can obviously see all the SSTEMS. They are there as fully as the performer.

Functioning as a double helix, the Piano interrogates the SSTEMS's existence on the stage and in the audience's minds. Together this discussion informs the artist so that their endeavors can match the scale of the medium. As I worked within this laboratory it became apparent that the performer/director/choreographer's comprehension and attitudes toward the audience was vitally important and influential to the type of work the artist could conceive of making. As I developed the practices of Presence work, the Dog-Sniff-Dog theory came into focus and indeed everything that was already in the Practice Manual took on a more fascinating aspect. I have found that the more you can acknowledge the audiences' capacity to understand, the greater are your designs in art. This shift from the stage to the audience's point of view offers the artist the possibility of interrogating their own intentions. This perspective removes the onus of pandering to the audiences and allows us to address the element of the audience as part of the creative process in performance.

This laboratory abruptly manifested itself in my studio on the fourth floor of 530 Canal Street. Laurie Anderson was in her loft on the sixth floor composing music and Pooh Kay was on the fourth floor choreographing and making films. It was early fall and I was feeling uncharacteristically satisfied with my life, my work, teaching and choreographing. I was quietly celebrating the accomplishment of my discovery of the SSTEMS. I was cavorting, waving my arms and playing with space, time, shapes, movements, logic, and my presence for no other reason than that they existed and I knew it. Suddenly I turned around in my mind and was imagining the audience. I paused, transfixed by the thought. Suddenly I realized that I had completed only half of the theory, and my heart sank. How could I manage to address the factor of the audience? I remember that I avoided the studio for days, overwhelmed and pissed off at having run into such an overwhelming question.

After some days of agonizing over this huge new blank territory, I was hurriedly crossing the floor of my studio, avoiding the Space, Shape Time, Emotion, Movement, Stories and the huge question in there, when the studio "stage" began to rise up, the floor lifting like the cover of a book or trap door, and fell over, covering the blank space, the "audience." What had just happened? Hanging at the apron of the stage, the SSTEMS had come up folded over onto the audience. Transfixed by the picture I began to realize that the SSTEMS existed as fully in the audience as they do onstage.

This picture would unfold a myriad of new perspectives and formations. I began to walk around my studio using my space lens but this time seeing what I was doing from the perspective of the audience. I lifted my arm and inspected my hand and saw the audience see my hand, then I saw the audience see me seeing my hand and realized that these spectators/participants were very good. If I thought of them as not good then what was I doing making dances for them? They were as good as I was. They had the capacity to see everything I wanted to show them and even things I did not consciously know I was showing them. I realized they were the finest pianos in the world. The audience, in this laboratory, became an instrument I could work with rather than a negative and frightening judge, or an ignorant, somewhat dangerous and demanding force.

Strengthened by this new laboratory and its perspective, in 1989 I finally refused to teach my usual composition/choreography class at ETW on the basis that the students did not have any time to work in studios by themselves in order to find what they cared about, and so had nothing to focus their creativity. These conditions seemed to me to engender mediocrity. Instead I came up with the idea that each student needed to try to find what was important to them as artists, and if they could do this we could start to make choreographic experiments. To set them in that direction I asked them to begin by establishing the belief that they had an audience for their work, an adoring audience who was waiting for the next big thing to come from them. The assignment was worded in this way. "Find your Perfect Audience and make a three-minute piece for them."

In the light of this focus I was amazed to find that audiences were often either ignored or thought of negatively as ignorant, less insightful, moody, perhaps unwilling to be there in general and or to extend themselves in a positive manner, insensitive to subtlety and experimentation, bullies prone to being judgmental and condemning, set in their ways, demanding only types of art that were familiar, and on the brink of going to sleep the minute the lights went down in the house. These were in part or in whole privately kept beliefs by performance makers that surfaced when I asked them to believe in an audience that believed in them.

On the inside they were not disposed to think of the audience as a very appealing part of the theater. This seemed justified. When you try to understand theater audiences from the standpoint of being your judge they can certainly look intimidating and unappealing. And then so it goes in reverse as well. If they are not appealing to you then you must not be that appealing to them. Then follows the idea that getting them to attend means promising them that they are going to see the show of the century, a spectacle they would not want to miss! Once they were seated it was absolutely important to make sure they did not go to sleep, so performance had to be broader, louder, and simpler than what they were expecting. Even if this psychology may not wholly define a performer's attitude, it can lurk beneath the surface in the studio. As performers struggled to wipe these negativities away they were in fact redefining the work conditions of their profession.

In the end each student came up with a small performance. I decided to not hold the usual critique and instead needed each student to describe their Perfect Audience. In other words, as audience, what did the performer/maker think we liked? In a class of 16 students there were 14 radically different audiences! We uncovered the startling information that there are extremely diverse reasons why performers, directors and choreographers are drawn to theater and dance. There is no singular definition of theater or dance because each person has a unique vision.

Reaching back into history for examples of performers who had special understanding of their audience I think of Marlon Brando, who was one of the most commanding and confident actors in communicating with the audience. His understanding of our perceptive ability allowed him to "exist" on film as much as he acted. He is hanging out with us, at times watching the movie with us; then he flips back and becomes the actor acting his role, then back to us. There is a "doubleness" to his performance that includes the audience in everything he does. This awareness is evident in On the Waterfront, and is visible all the way to The Godfather.

In the postmodern dance scene, one of my great inspirations has been the choreographer/dancer Yvonne Rainer. She seems to understand the microscopic absorptive ability of her audiences. My first encounter was when I watched her perform as a member of the Grand Union dance group on an outdoor plaza in San Francisco in the late sixties. Most of her performance involved her reading a book in front of the audience. Much as I wanted to watch all the other excellent performers, I could not keep my eyes off her. When you absolutely know what you want to try, and trust the audience to extend themselves to reach out to you—that is, trust the perceptual abilities of your audience—you have tremendous authority. In more recent times, Johnny Depp seems to play with his audience to such a degree that it sometimes seems like he is not actually in the movie plot so much as just directly goofing around with those who are watching him. He works his magic on us through his strange timing, his amazingly creative postures and spatial choices. His is a three-hundred-and-sixty-degree acting technique, done with the confidence that we can see every nuance of his work.

I tell my students that they must define their audience, work on their Piano, know it and understand how to play what they want on it as well as they possibly can. I define my audiences as being incredibly sensitive, perceptive of my very breathing and thoughts. Others can define the audience as rowdy, course, liking bad jokes and there for a good time. The definitions of your audience seem infinitely various to me.

CHAPTER 13

The Matrix

The Ingredients Are in the Cauldron

AS THE PERFORMANCE TECHNIQUE, THE SIX VIEWPOINTS IS A MATRIX of performed Space, Shape, Time, Emotion, Movement and Story. The performer is immersed within the physical presence of the languages of the SSTEMS. The Matrix laboratory is formed of the physical natural phenomena of the materials. When performance practice evolves, the SSTEMS become available in every moment onstage. This matrix-like perspective evolves from the origin focus on one material at a time. This eventually instills a perceptual nimbleness; simultaneously the performer is aware of:

- the visual impact
- temporal play
- shape options
- kinetics

- their presence
- the audience
- he narrative
- the philosophical roots

The Matrix is the laboratory of the fully functioning observer/participant Rather than approaching performance as the creator/originator, which requires that you distance yourself from creative work, the observer/participant performer stands within the materials allowing them ot direct action as equal partners.

CURRICULUM 11

THE MATRIX

Working in the Matrix we begin to experience that each of the six materials has sub-properties that form complex links. These intersections make it possible to choose at any moment a new direction for your perceptions. In reassembling theater from this subtle and nonhierarchical place, we are working inside a matrix of the subtlest interaction of the parts:

My advanced students and many of my own choreographies have drawn from the interrelationships found in the following:

Space can dialogue with Shape: *dictating the types of shapes and where to place them*

Space can dialogue with Time: *radically changing the awareness of the passage of time*

Space can dialogue with Emotion: *causing elation or fear, expansion or violence*

Space can dialogue with Movement: *suggesting large patters or tiny gestures*

Space can dialogue with Story: *capable of holding history or eradicating it*

Shape can dialogue with Space: *a vase can demand the dimensions of a room it prefers*

Shape can dialogue with Time: *round shapes are slower than angular*

Shape can dialogue with Emotion: *softness, harshness, accepting, rejecting*

Shape can dialogue with Movement: *a shape can dictate kinetic possibilities*

Shape can dialogue with Story: *a stooped spine or foot on point can be the main plot*

To understand this phenomenological study of the nature of the stage and performance, you cannot just read about it. You must actively experience it. The word "matrix" comes from the Latin, which means a situation or surrounding substance within which something else originates, develops, or is contained.

On my route from 530 Canal Street to NYU, I cross several huge roadways—Hudson Street, Seventh Avenue, Sixth Avenue—then I enter SoHo on Spring Street, turn up West Broadway, cross Houston Street into the West Village, cross the park Washington Square, slip inside the door to the Tisch Building and up a flight of steps and I am in the studios about to face hungry students.

The route is like a double pressure zone. I love the emptiness and industrial indifference but there is a kind of unspoken pressure that hovers inside SoHo. People are discovered, we are all under a new kind of scrutiny, scrambling to keep up with our new more public images. The responsibilities that we create and shouldered are turning into other people's business. Reviewers, producers, gallery owners—the public is watching and following.

My memory of the arrival of the Matrix hovers over this route because for the year or more I traveled it, dodging trucks, I was dangerously preoccupied with the problem of how to codify an emerging three-dimensional manifestation of the SSTEMS. Teetering on my bicycle, riding past Richard Nonas's studio and the Wooster Group's Performing Garage, thinking of all the artists around me working so hard, gathering in the strength of their visions, their process, and their outcomes, I prayed that I could find a way to impart my developing philosophy. I thought of drawing it, and tried, but came up with an almost solid black cube from all the lines I drew depicting the SSTEMS interacting with each other. The drawing looked like a Richard Serra but it was not communicating what I needed it to.

There was an isolated auto parts store on Hudson Street. I once went in to look for a valve for my Ford Falcon. At the counter I saw a book with transparent pages that overlaid each other forming pictures of my car's engine. After seeing it I kept obsessing about making a book of transparencies depicting the SSTEMS in all their interrelatedness but finally gave it up and waited in the usual blank space for something

(continued)

CURRICULUM 11: *THE MATRIX* (continued)

The following iterations are for you to investigate on your own:

Time can dialogue with Space
Time can dialogue with Shape
Time can dialogue with Emotion
Time can dialogue with Movement
Time can dialogue with Story

Emotion can dialogue with Space
Emotion can dialogue with Shape
Emotion can dialogue with Time
Emotion can dialogue with Movement
Emotion can dialogue with Story

Movement can dialogue with Space
Movement can dialogue with Shape
Movement can dialogue with Time
Movement can dialogue with Emotion
Movement can dialogue with Story

Story can dialogue with Space
Story can dialogue with Shape
Story can dialogue with Time
Story can dialogue with Emotion
Story can dialogue with Movement

to come rescue me. This was 1980 and on March 31, 1999, Hollywood finally rescued me. *The Matrix* premiered in movie theaters across the nation.

As we approach the Matrix of the Six Viewpoints, it would be good to go back to walking. This simple action is such an enduring touchstone for the Viewpoints actor.

ACTOR: Where are we?

THE MATRIX: You are back in the studio, pacing back and forth practicing Walking and Stopping in Space, but now you are also aware of the possibilities contained in the Piano Laboratory and of reifying the existence of all six materials simulta- neously. Now as you perform Walking and Stopping you are able to practice the skill of focusing on one, two, or all of the SSTEMS, and include the audience in your practice. Your resources have expanded in the microscopic, quiet, "turn things upside down and inside out" world of deconstruction.

ACTOR: This sounds a little unstable, technical, undramatic and unemotional.

THE MATRIX: Think of a peculiar pair of glasses. Let's call these the Six Viewpoints glasses. The frames are fitted with six pairs of lenses. Each lens filters out five of the materials and pulls up only the one you want to work with. The lenses are six awarenesses. The performer can flip from lens to lens or combine lenses making more subtle actions. The Viewpoints Matrix extends performing as a suspended mixture of Time, Shape, Space, Movement, Emotion and Story with the ease that Keanu Reeves dodges bullets in the The Matrix.

ACTOR: Wow. That is quite a claim.

THE MATRIX: This Viewpoints Matrix process is equal to the Stanislavski Method of sense memory. Sense memory is a method of reaching into the actor's past experience to find a key that will stimulate the desired emotion required by a specific character in a scene. This practice of sense memory is a very sophisticated technique that gave theater a great jolt. More depth, and more fluid reality was suddenly onstage, pouring off the stage, engaging the audience in a simulation of life. With this technique so much more could be communicated. The art of acting took a giant step forward.

Actor: So this Matrix thing is equal to Stanislavski?

The Matrix: Equal and very different. The Six Viewpoints Matrix is similar to sense memory in its ability to deliver more diverse action onto the stage. In some ways it too shakes up the status quo, yet comes from a totally different source and perspective. The ability to change lenses, to be performing in Shape and then flip to Story throws the activity of acting and actions into a much more multidimensional field of play.

The performer has six powerful sources of action. In real life we act in these languages subconsciously anyway: you might be talking about how much money is in your bank account; pause fleetingly to fill your mind with the pattern and design of the carpet on the floor of the bank; shift focus to the dress you put on this morning; suddenly stop, as unattended time passes by—then experience a sudden explosion of very physical movement trying to bring your attention back to the moment by waking up your body.

CURRICULUM 12

FLIPPING LENSES

Try it. Are you still walking? Good. Begin walking in a fairly large circle. As you walk, try flipping lenses. Pull up your Shape lens; sud- denly you are aware of the position of your arms, the changing of your feet, the carriage of your head. Now switch lenses to Space. Now you are aware of the room, and the circle you are inscribing in the room becomes the focus of your performance. You begin to project this spatial pattern to the audience and then you switch to Time. Is it pedestrian in nature? Is it going to slide into a kind of even march? Is the Time you are in designed to soothe and relax the audience? Here you are beginning to float in six separate realities, choosing one then another, buoyant, flexible, and acutely aware of performing.

This is real life flipping from one lens to another.

Let us take a closer look at a Viewpoints actor: Oh, I see her over there standing in the studio—she is still in her blue jeans; she forgot her sweat pants. She just came from her day job. She may not be able to keep it together to always bring her sweats, but there is this very dressed-down look to her body. Even the ritual clothing for rehearsal is not necessary for her anymore. She has a kind of blank willingness to do—to do anything. Her presence is loose and luminous from the attention and love that she has come to understand is her right.

Through the particalization-like focuses of her movement training, she knows how to share her physical life with other human beings. Some of this ability has come from her studies of Contact Improvisation, and the ever-present rolling on the floor. This was not easy for her to achieve. For a long time she did not like being lifted, supporting others, or rolling on the floor. She felt that her hips were too large, and she really was not comfortable being touched all over. It took about three years to get this skill together, and as she did, she came to love and understand her body and this made it possible to embrace the SSTEMS. Her body changed from being some foreign, obstinate object to being a system that included a vast performance instrument.

Presence became much easier for her. She discovered, in one session of Walking and Stopping, that she loved communicating with Space and seemed to have a talent for seeing theater from a visual point of view. Each of the Viewpoints practices had its revelations, and now they stick with her no matter what she is attempting to do.

CHAPTER 14

Doing the Unnecessary Laboratory

The SSTEMS Dissolve

A SMALL FLAT, ROUND STONE IS SKIMMED ALONG THE SURFACE OF A quiet pond. It hits the surface and jumps off, hits again, rises, hits again, and again, and again. The pond is theater, the stone is tossed by my youthful self, in my excited engagement with performance. Each time the stone strikes represents a small work of performance I did as a child, each causing a desperate need for more information about what I was trying to do. As the stone skims and bounces I am beginning to realize that I must come to know theater and dance, the medium of performance as whole, in its technical entirety if possible. I want to know it like painters know painting on a technical level.

These last concentric circles undulate across the pond's surface: The Matrix, Doing the Unnecessary, and the Original Anarchist. The conclusions of our journey, these three laboratories, provide a creative self-affirmation. They speak of the arrival of a Viewpoints-prepared theater artist, evolved and set into action by the preceding chapters.

Oh good, they all have their sweatpants on. They will surely need them—things are going to get messy. Doing the Unnecessary is just what its name infers: the task of interfering with ordinary, automatic actions such as walking, speaking, reaching, exiting, entering, taking off our coat, or sitting down. We are going to ask the performers to reverse all the careful, delicate, subtle training they have been receiving throughout this book. *Halt! Drop your training and step away. If I observe you using any minimal/efficient coordination, proper spatial judgment, appro- priate timing, or readable gestures, you will be severely punished: I will drop you back into the flat hierarchical world.*

Whether trained in Viewpoints or any other technique actors normally "rest" in the necessary. They produce efficient, coordinated, meaningful actions either in a hierarchical structure or a nonhierarchical structure. They are able to use the correct timing they intend when they speak, the right amount of muscle to perform movements, the right shapes to sit, stand, hold a coffee cup, the right spatial judgments so they can walk through doorways and avoid bumping into the other actors. They embody the "correct" emotions, and they keep their stories/ logic straight.

For all of us this training started at birth and has proceeded sequentially until this well planned achievement results in . . . oh no, I can't bear to say it! . . . desensitizing us. Ahhh! How are we going to be fully awakened when what we are actually doing out of habit is numbing our senses? Half-asleep in these efficient actions, the body and mind begin to be not fully present.

> **PERFORMERS:** Desensitized!? What are you talking about? First you claim
> we are getting sensitized by dialoguing with the materials, and now you
> are exclaiming that we must reach beyond the SSTEMS because they too
> can contain an element of desensitizing actions?

Until now my classroom was unusually quiet for a theater training class. The sun pours in the windows and we quietly walk and walk, or stare at our limbs, or sit while others watch us; we try executing various unusual times and read in our reading circles. The materials are met in contemplation.

Sound odd? Yes. Yes it is. In this chaos our Awakened Actor's body/mind connections are on high alert. They are easing into what I call "tiger mode." The brain synapses are firing at a much higher rate than normal; they are becoming animal and more. Their eyes are able to focus and register distance with astonishing accuracy, the hand reaches out to catch the chair leg, to catch the shoe as it flies by, and they can still concentrate on the removal of an arm from the sleeve of someone else's shirt. Certainly no one is asleep in this room. They have walked into the crazy world of Art, wide open creativity, no boundaries, no meaning, no consequences.

I have seen many classes use impulse work to train acuity. For me the problem with this work is that needs to traverse a painful stretch of self-consciousness. The break into reflexive response, thorough impulse work is often very brief—exciting, but brief. It does not take the brain very long to catch up and begin to reflect rather than to just do.

In the world of Doing the Unnecessary, as we glide toward the end of our journey, the actors open the door to not-knowing and, by doing this, revel in the delight of broken intention, hyperawake in the mad tossup of an un-reified art world. They are at the very edge of exploration, without any responsibility to anything. What a relief! Something is being restored. In this stratosphere of Doing the Unnecessary, the body is released to its own wonderful knowledge unattended. Our physical/ mental self is uninhibited by perspective, contemplation, or reflection.

Aside from the acceleration in the speed of brain synapses (always a good thing), the performer finds that art/creativity becomes a different world filled with oxygen. The traditional creator/originator, who must take on the bone-crushing, challenging task of generating a new idea is replaced by this swinging, casual, hang-loose inhabitant of the Unnecessary. In this finishing school, a maturity comes. An acceptance arrives, and they understand that they are surrounded by and filled with wonderful stuff. The Six Viewpoints say their task is just to develop the skill to recognize what is there and put it to use. But for a truly awakened artist it is also absolutely important as an extension to swing with the incidental and the accidental, to take up the butterfly net and go out hunting.

CURRICULUM 13

DOING THE UNNECESSARY

Now the performers stand ready to turn the room into a nuclear fision reactor! They are going to spend the afternoon trying not to know how to walk, or how to do anything they might normally do. They are going to miss going through the door!

Suddenly her limbs are all twisted up and he is trying to turn the doorknob with his feet. While opening the door, he is being given a new hairstyle by a classmate who is using a shoe, shoelace, and sock to accomplish this grooming procedure. No one in the room is doing any- thing that anyone else would expect them to do. Having gotten the door open, he exits to the hall but cannot close the door because he has not removed his left hand from the room. Someone decides that this hand is a convenient hook for their coat—and unfortunately, they have not removed their coat. Our actress manages to get partway across the room and is sitting on a chair that is turned upside down. I usually allow this practice to continue for a hour or hour and a half. It is important to experience that there are limitless resources in the Unnecessary.

CHAPTER 15

The Original Anarchist

A New and Very Old Idea

HERE AT THE END OF THE SIX VIEWPOINTS, WE HAVE TRAVERSED EIGHT laboratories and have come to know the SSTEMS from so many different perspectives. We have seen them in microscopic detail and macroscopic applications. Emerging from the finishing school of the gracious and delightful Unnecessary Laboratory, our shoes and socks back on our feet, we can all take a break and go to dinner. We have no more work for the time being because our journey has transformed us. We are now Original Anarchists.

> **PERFORMER:** What does it mean to be an Original Anarchist? Why do you call me that? Why is that where the whole practice and theory end?

> **SIX VIEWPOINTS:** An Original Anarchist is one who is deeply familiar with Space, Shape, Time, Emotion, Movement and Story. One who knows inches and empti- ness, being, the toss of a stone and the tensing of a muscle and the significance of language and memory, how to find one's way to the Experimental Theatre Wing at 721 Broadway, New York, New York, 10012 . . . blood, mud, pulse, gravity, water, weight, sensation.

> **PERFORMER:** I thought an anarchist was a person who is against the rules and laws of society?

Six Viewpoints: That is the second idea of what an anarchist is. That definition of anarchist started in the 18th century to identify groups and artists who were against organized society. The original definition is subtly but radically different: one who is directly connected with nature and needs no outside rules as guides in order to function as a positive part of the whole.

Let us take a look at our Six Viewpoints Original Anarchists. They have been following instructions, yet the Six Viewpoints calls them anarchists. How could this be? They have meekly walked in Space when commanded to do so. They have measured rooms obeying the laws of mathematics. They have toiled in the Matrix, studiously holding their attention to the multiple dialogues of Space, Shape, Time, Emotion, Movement and Story—the SSTEMS. They are now very proud that they have completed the Bridge and worked with the materials in a philosophical, conceptual, and practical system of Viewpoints particalization. So you see, they are not really anti-law, anti-system, or anti-rules as would be an anarchist in the commonly understood, modern definition.

The rules they know are ones learned from the circumstances of their interactions with the SSTEMS and the Laboratories. They are one with the movement of their blood, beginning to be expert at playing with the forces of gravity, comforted by their subtle awareness of the presence of the human being. The rules established by these forces do not have to be rejected because they are not imposed. When our performer acquires a deep knowledge of the laws of gravity, sensation, central nervous system, logic, form, geometry, etc. they have developed an awesome sense of self-affirmation. The importance of this focus is emblematic of the revolution in dance and in theater that took place many years ago but can still be seen in ever greater expansion today.

This Six Viewpoints training, and the work of many artists who are working in similar modes of deconstruction, brings artists uniquely close to action in the fullest sense of the word. This closeness, established by walking in Space, dialoguing with Shape, sensing Movement, living in Time, results in performers who rely on their own judgment; confident enough to wait until the positive ideas or action are clear;

able to be generous; able to interact on a vast variety of planes of communication. We now see performers who are able to be cooperative without being locked into an arbitrary unity; we see action that is diverse in focus and tempo and complexity. I cannot say for sure, but it seems to me that the quality of performance today in films, stage, choreography and music is so much richer than it has ever been. And this in turn allows the audience to be more intelligent in the use of their senses and their concepts of the world around them. Did this early revolution cause what is happening how? It is impossible to say. What is clear is that it is part of the continuum of development that we see today in the performing arts.

These qualities of independence, courage, confidence, and cooperation are often unseen accumulative results of our journey through the Laboratories with the SSTEMS. What has happened? I am going to ask our actress to come back to work for us one last time so we can glimpse the effects of having become an Original Anarchist.

As she takes up the microscopic focus of News of a Difference, in this conceptual and practical engagement, she is beyond the judgment of good actress/bad actress, ingénue/character actress, etc. Her involvement with this Laboratory quietly lures her eye to the periphery of the stage. She establishes an awareness of a downstage-left lighting pole. There it stands, only two inches from one of the velvety curtain wings, the cold tension of its black metal presence and its placement embodying a kind of intriguing secretiveness. It feels interesting to be engaged with something that is essentially a secret onstage. As she walks over to it and stands between the curtain and the metal, she discovers that an absolute refuge is formed there in the gap between the two. The communion of the two surfaces beckons her to stay awhile. Then she walks out into the vast space of the stage floor and then, by another route, returns to the small space.

She is becoming aware of an odd thought, the possibility of hiding on stage. Why not? What a wonderful, vivid, human activity. Hidden, she can watch the audience. By doing this she is turning the theater around on itself and exposing a rarely examined possibility in the role of an actress, in the possibilities of acting. She is feeling a new kind of power with the idea that she can hide on stage, have secrets and observe the audience as a part of theater. Is she a good actress? Who knows? She is certainly deeply engaged. And that is one of the great bases of acting. She emerges from this rehearsal with a patina of the Original Anarchist gleaming in her presence, through her eyes and in her manner. She has used the process of contemplation, and is aware of having exposed a wealth of information.

Instead of taking a break and going out to eat, as suggested, our young man has spent the last hour improvising with the SSTEMS. He feels an odd mixture of vulnerability and invulnerability. He makes things without anyone telling him what to do, or even telling himself what to do. At some point in the session he found reason to fall to the floor, but once there, he decides to deconstruct this line of action and to re-reify what he is doing. He decides to become the anchor. He just stays where he is., motionless. It is a beautiful effect; suddenly, because of the stillness of his action, the stage becomes full of awareness.

Through this the Horizontal starts oozing into the room more powerfully by his act of stillness and changing of focus. His deconstruction brings about a condition in which the audience is allowed to become equal to the performer because they are both engaged in the activity of observer/participant with the materials.

As his feelings of vulnerability and invulnerability hover over his work they are secured by his understanding that he has just physically and philosophically engaged in the Laboratory of Postmodernism. He understands that he is side-stepping the rules of Modernism and a creative hierarchy which gave the director or choreographer the authority of authorship. He knows that he is in a horizontal, nonhierarchical relationship to the stage, the audience and to creativity. This he knows directly relates him to the process and voice of our time: a sense of knowledge and formation of systems that are free-floating in cyberspace and in the studio.

Both performers will be one of the reifiers of this new type of training and perspective if they continue down this path. They know that they articulate and thereby verify the process and viability of rethinking, rearticulating, and reshaping the future. Their time in the Laboratories has leveled the playing field of theater by defining the audience and the artist as similarly endowed entities who understand, feel and speak the same language. As young Original Anarchists they can look their audience square in the eyes. They are not afraid of complexity at any level. After all, their acting techniques are part of the Matrix!

By the time this last Laboratory came about, I had given up hope of ever finishing the Six Viewpoints. In fact I did not know that it was possible to finish a theory. When it was finished I could not speak for several days. I was experiencing a phenomenon. I had thrown a small stone into a pond. The stone was a question: "What is theater made of?" Now the ensuing ripples reached the edge of the pond and were coming back, one by one, to melt into stillness again. To express this I found myself taking my wrist in my mouth to from a kind of circle. Someone commented that this looked like the ouroboros, the snake biting its own tail, a symbol from ancient Greek culture.

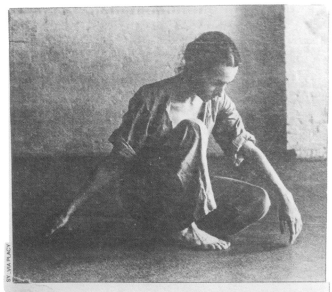

SY_VIA PLACY

Mary Overlie: Enigmatic Witness

By Sally R. Sommer

One hot day last summer, a cluster of peo
ple lounged on the street and sidewalk of
West Broadway, watching Mary Overlie per
form in a display window of Holly Solomon's
gallery. She was suspended, waiting in a re
laxed arabesque, her arms draped over her
head. Then the head slipped out of the encir
cling arms and tilted slightly, while the arms
still cradled the shape of a head no longer
there. Highly sensitized, she seemed to be
listening for a secret signal we could never
hear. Then movement. An explosion of trem
bling begins in the foot, coursing through the
leg and torso, finally flying out of the finger
tips of one hand. Our eyes fastened back on
Overlie's face: She has remained calmly gaz
ing at—seeming to think about—the foot
that initiated this rush of movement.

She has a curious way of splitting concen
tration, of presenting *herself*, which is utterly
compelling. As she dances, she watches what
she does, rather like an unruffled, nonjudg
mental witness. Actor David Warrilaw, of
Mabou Mines, has compared this watchful
ness to "Grotowski's idea of the 'silent part
ner,' or witnessing in the Buddhist sense, or
the artist's eye—movement filtered through
consciousness."

Overlie—who is presenting a new work,
Painters Dream, at the Kitchen June 8 to
10—describes the process as holding a per
sonal score of images in her mind, sometimes
emotional, sometimes spatial, and these men
tal pictures cause the movement to bubble
up. Watching her dance, I feel a double and
equal involvement. The images imbue the
movement with emotion that remains com
pletely enigmatic. But its intensity is tem
pered because it rebounds against her own
quiet observation. I do not know what those
images are, nor is it important, nor do I sus
pect they remain the same for each perfor
mance of a dance. David Warrilaw per
formed that same summer day in her piece.
He stood alone in a window smoking, chat
ting, blowing his nose, his dance an accumu
lation of gestures both funny and forlorn.
Framed and behind glass, we could hear
nothing of what he said, the emotional over
lay intense and disturbing because it was
grounded in what was for us a silent text. In
order to fuse what was seen with what was
felt, the mind tended to create its own sce
nario, to conjure up its own private score of
associations, the more powerful because they
were so personal. Overlie puts her dances
together in such a way that the audience is se
duced into participation, entering the land
scapes of our own minds, and two sets of pri
vate images mesh in public performance.

Village Voice review by Sally R. Sommer, 1978.

Village Voice review, 1978 (continued)

She has choreographed dances for odd spaces. Holly Solomon's windows provided a stage eight feet high, two feet deep, and five feet wide. At another performance, five dancers were compressed in one window, dressed in muted green, the slight imperfections and quivering of the glass lending the dance an eerie underwater quality, movement rippling through the group like currents. The year before she made a dance on an indoor football field for Lee Breuer's (Mabou Mines) *The Saint and the Football Player*. Thirty dancers wheeled about in huge patterns, then slowly fell onto a mound of crumpled bodies, which were scooped up in the jaws of five fork lifts. The bodies draped and fell from the raising prongs, and as the machines moved forward, they left a path littered with human debris.

JoAnne Akalaitis's *Dressed Like an Egg* had a dance by Overlie, placed on a Mylar runner stretched across the width of the stage. A half-curtain cut the performers off above the knees, so all focus centered on the feet. The women wore clear plastic shoes, the hollow high heels glimmering with tiny lights. This dance was a gentle, witty seduction of light taps, pattering out a Morse Code of love. Gradually, the women's feet were joined by men's feet in dapper shoes. A duet, a brief engagement. Then four pairs of shoes began a waltzing flirtation, the women's shoes attached to the arms of the men.

David Warrilaw has described Overlie's work with actors as being tremendously compassionate. She doesn't impose her dance on them but elicits a style of movement that is their own, weaving it into the pattern of the dance. When she teaches she does the same thing, and it reminds me of a statement that an early modern dancer, Loie Fuller, made in 1909. She said that she did not teach her "children," that they were not learning, but *attaining*.

Overlie is investigating performance presence in her work, that elusive quality everyone instantly recognizes and no one defines well. Because she does not use narrative or character or tasks—nor is she interested in personality—what remains is the investigation of self through a distillation of personal images expressed in movement. It is revealing and baffling. Presence cannot be called up without something else going on, a deeply involved concentration concurrent with activity.

Although she is clear and direct in conversation, when discussing her work she evokes the same paradox of calm simplicity and intense inner complexity so characteristic of her dancing. I find myself reverting to my own associations, or reaching for someone else's impressions (such as Warrilaw's) in an attempt to explain the power of her presence as person and performer. ∎

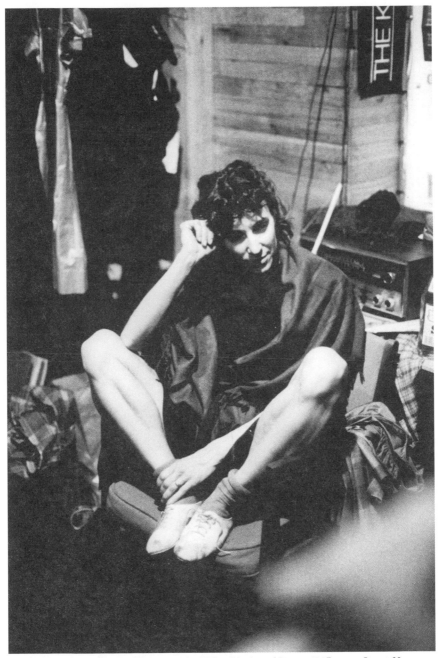

Overlie backstage at The Kitchen Center for Video, Music and Dance, 484 Broome Street, New York City.

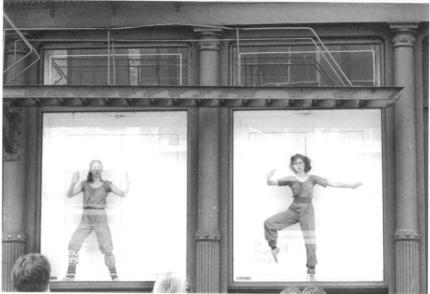

Glass Imagination I, Holly Solomon Gallery on West Broadway, 1976. Left: Mary Overlie Right: Margaret Eginton. Photographer: Theo Robinson.

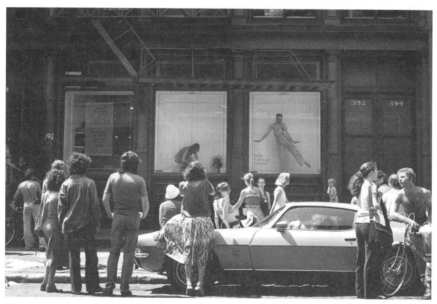

Glass Imagination II, Holly Solomon Gallery on West Broadway, 1977. Left window: Jan Wenk; Right window: Mary Overlie. Photographer: Theo Robinson.

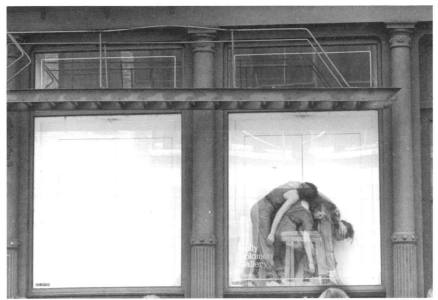

Glass Imagination I, Holly Solomon Gallery on West Broadway, 1976. Left to right: Danny Lepkoff, Margaret Eginton, Dan Hurlan. Photographer: Theo Robinson.

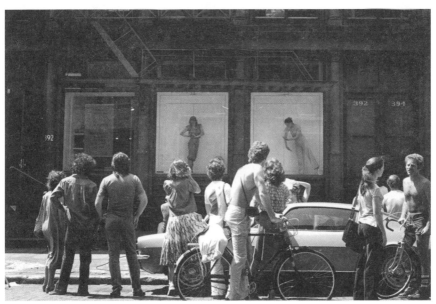

Glass Imagination II, Holly Solomon Gallery on West Broadway, 1977. Left window: Jan Wenk; Right window: Mary Overlie. Photographer: Theo Robinson.

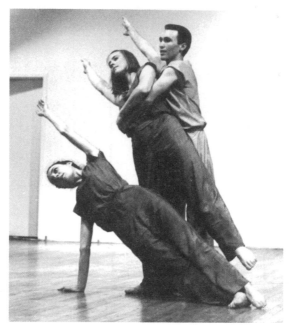

Hero, The Kitchen Center for Video, Music and Dance, 484 Broome Street, 1979. Left to right: Mary Overlie, Nina Martin, Wendell Beavers.

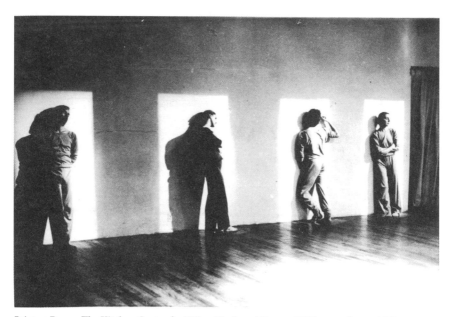

Painters Dream, The Kitchen Center for Video, Music and Dance, 484 Broome Street, 1978. Left to right: Paul Langland, Nina Martin, Wendell Beavers, Mary Overlie.

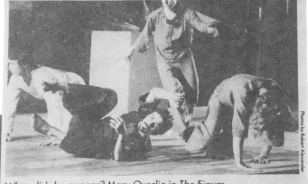

CONCEPTS IN PERFORMANCE

When did she appear? Mary Overlie in *The Figure*

The Soho Weekly News Oct. 26, 1978

Mary Overlie's *The Figure* continues her interest in the ways visual arts and dance reveal the human body. Waiting for the dance to begin out in the museum garden, watching people walking inside the building, noticing the huge canvases with Overlie's reclining figure drawn on them in blue outline, suddenly I saw Overlie lying on a platform, dressed in blue, in one of the poses in the drawings. When did she appear? I noticed her for a while, comparing her form and mass to the drawings. And then three other dancers had appeared, in darker blue, yellow, red. They rolled, ran, crossed the space in a clump, compressing their individual spaces yet seeming to cleave open the space around the group. They kept the group so closely knit that they always seemed tangled in each other's bodies, nearly colliding as they dropped to the ground, got up, moved swiftly.

Suddenly the other three froze as Overlie danced alone, balancing softly, her arms outstretched, her breath audible. Movements of the arms and legs brought her body out of control. There was a sudden flurry of small gestural details, coming in clots, punctuated by stillnesses. Meanwhile, the others had changed their positions. But I hadn't seen them move. The events pressed me to be aware of how I notice change and motion. Overlie casually walked away and the dance was over. ●

The Soho Weekly News, review of *The Figure,* performed at the Museum of Modern Art Summer Garden,1978. Photographer: Robert Alexander.

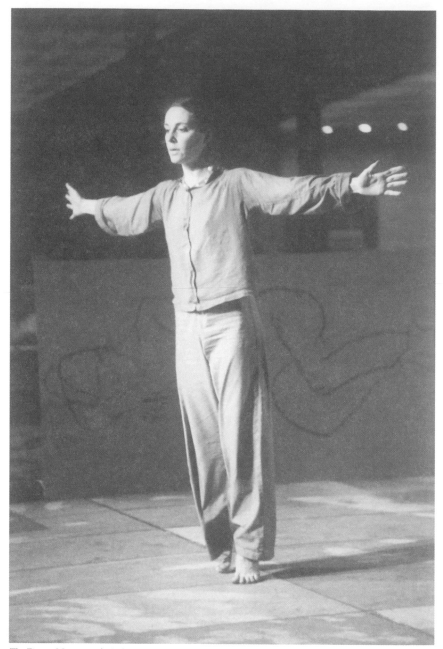

The Figure, Museum of Modern Art Summer Garden, 1978. Mary Overlie. Photographer: Robert Alexander.

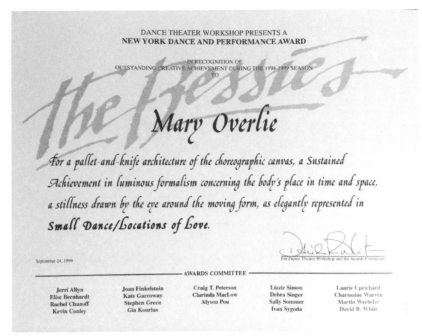

Bessie Award, 1999.

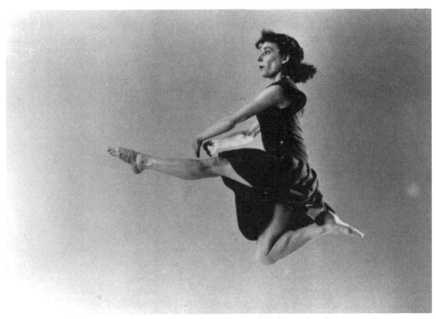

History, The Kitchen Center for Video, Music and Dance, 1983. Mary Overlie.

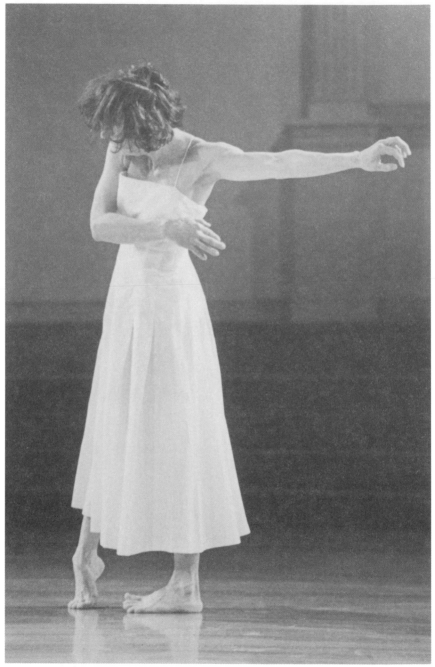

Location of Love/Small Dance, Danspace at St. Mark's Church, 1998. Mary Overlie.

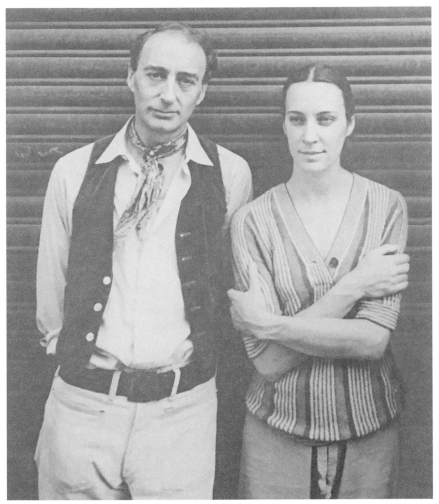

Actor David Warrilow (a founding member of Mabou Mines Theater Company) and Mary Overlie, West Broadway, circa 1978.

PART THREE

THE
PRACTICE MANUAL

The Viewpoints Basic Practices

SEPARATION IS AT THE ROOT OF ALL TECHNICAL DEVELOPMENT. IN the practice of Japanese ink drawing, the breath, mind, body, brush and ink are first separated and then recombined to guarantee maximum freedom of articulation to each part and to the whole. It is more difficult for artists in the theater to see this process because we have such a long history of being told that it should all flow from the unconscious, or "naturally." In this regard, Postmodernism has been a great influence on the theater. In the past, with ideas still stacked up in a vertical hierarchy, it was difficult to attain structural freedom. With the exception of the last few "advanced practices" all the practices in this manual have been in place as my teaching method since 1983. They have received a great deal of polishing over the years.

As you approach these practices, remember that the rules are designed to make it possible to separate the Viewpoints from each other. Mobility can be achieved from focusing on a single Viewpoint, or SSTEMS, at a time. To achieve this avoid the usual hierarchical habit of combining materials in order to feel that you are "making art," "getting somewhere," or accomplishing something. For instance, start with achieving a true knowledge of Space before you let yourself mix it with Time, Shape, Movement, Emotion, or Story. Separate and focus; combining can always happen later. Work slowly at first. The slower you go the deeper you get. Ah, time!

Space Practices

Practice 1: Walking and Stopping in Space

Solo and group practice

Setting up the practice: Using walking and stopping, focus on exploring the space.

Slowly develop familiarity and facility with space through observing the practice room as you change perspective by walking and stopping. Observe your spatial placement in relationship to the walls of the room and to the other performers. All paths, formations and positions will gradually become vocabularies. Explore the dimensions of the floor space, the distance between walls, and the distance between people, the visual angles and placement of performers; begin to know space through feet and inches. Use your body to feel relationships.

Do not add movements beyond walking.

Do not add shapes to the body beyond its simplest form of standing.

Do not use time by falling into a rhythm, or focusing on how long you walk, or at what speed.

Allow yourself to sink into the dialogue set up by this practice.

Returning to this dialogue again and again reveals ever increasing information, especially if you use the principles of News of a Difference.

Benefit

This practice has a remarkable way of bringing a group of performers together in a consciously acknowledged spatial dialogue. Directors, choreographers, and improvisation companies can use this work to build a strong ensemble. Awareness of space develops peripheral vision, which in turn, improves awareness of other performers and the total look of the stage. Actors and dancers develop the ability to take and give focus. This practice also develops the awareness that the stage can magnify action and improves awareness of what the audience is seeing.

Practice 2: The Grid (conceived by Barbara Dilley)

Solo and group practice

Setting up the practice: Place an imaginary grid that covers the entire room. The grid must be fairly precise and steady.

Imagine that you are working on a piece of graph paper. It can help to place shoes or other objects at the end points of each line to keep the spacing, however this level of precision is not mandatory. At the beginning of the work on the grid the vocabulary should be strictly limited to walking and stopping. Movement along the grid must not be altered to allow passage. If you meet someone on your path you must stop and wait, back up or turn until you find another line that is free of obstruction. All movement must be found through a solution on the grid.

More Viewpoints can be added later as advanced studies, exploring Time, Shape, Movement, Story and Emotion in the special alterations of the original practice.

Benefit

This practice develops clarity of spatial positions. It is also an ensemble-building tool. Once you are able to see space though the structure of the grid it is easier to remember and execute floor patterns and blocking.

Practice 3: 1/4 Space

Begin this work as a solo exploration and expand to small groups of four to six, once the basic work becomes clear on an individual level.

Setting up the practice: Stand in the space and sense the flow of energy as it travels through the room. Allow this energy flow to move your body through space. In Group practice, the individuals endeavor to work as one unit comprised of individual elements. The focus must be to stay together balancing the pull of the energy paths against the focus on group cohesion.

All spaces have a spatial flow, paths, along which energy flows through the room. Allow your body to be carried or pushed by that flow. The flow can take you to the floor, roll you, lift you, hold you in one place. Do not move without the exterior suggestion of spatial flow.

The second step with this work is done in a group. The group should not be bigger than six to begin with. The group should extend their awareness to form one body. Keep the group as solid as possible while allowing the flow of spatial movement in the room to carry the group into motion.

This practice allows spatial energy to be explored as a conscious source of movement. It is very much like doing contact improvisation but with space instead of with another human being. I discovered the principle for the practice in a study of kung fu. That form uses the flow of energy in the space to carry the blow or avert your opponent's strike.

Benefit

Through this practice you can start to acquire space as a partner. Space becomes as real and dimensional as a script, music or another performer. This work also builds confidence in opening up to outside impulses that take the performer past their own auto-generated stance (which is so often taught in acting classes).

Practice 4: Architectural Space

Solo practice

Setting up the practice: Explore the walls, doors, windows, nails, boards, holes, pipes, light fixtures, etc. Attention should be drawn by interest and remain on the object of interest until one is satisfied. The object of your interest can be explored with the fingers, the mouth, the skin, the eyes, ears, etc.

It is necessary to feel that you have your entire life to go on looking at the space. This casual approach is very important especially the first few times it is done in a new space. As you work the space comes alive through your attention. Actors and dancers can begin to incorporate the strength of the architecture in performance. Do not project character or situation onto the architecture. If later on you want to create a fantasy will be stronger if you know how much real information there is in a curtain, chair or wall.

Perform solo and group architectural improvisations for the class

Benefit

This practice reveals how rich actual spaces can be, how much they can suggest on their own in terms of drama, framing and movement.

Practice 5: Near, Far and Infinite Space (inspired by Lisa Nelson)

Solo practice

We all have different natural engagements of space. I have discovered that our individual engagement of space falls into three general categories of spatial awareness and projections:

Near Space: references only the space that the body occupies Far Space: references the walls, floor and ceiling (the container)

Infinite Space: references beyond the boundaries of the theater, to the infinite.

Being aware of this individual definition and being able to modulate projection is a skill which can be developed. The ability to modulate spatial projection provides range and nuance.

The actor or dancer can appear self-contained, their body and movement highly visible when working in Near Space. The actor or dancer can metaphorically touch the walls of the theater when working in Far Space.

The actor of dancer can project off the planet when working in Infinite Space.

Setting up the practice: Practice walking on the stage or in the studio exploring your natural focus. Which are you, Near, Far or Infinite? Then explore what it is like to have your awareness in the other two that are not as accessible to you.

Benefit

This practice teaches that the idea of space can be projected. Being able to discriminate between the three focuses is very helpful in doing character work. This focus can be used in a more complex manner by setting up a scene or choreographer in which the characters or dancer is given a specific spatial focus. I have found that this vocabulary can also be helpful as a dramaturgical tool in interpreting the work of the playwright by analyzing whether their characters are expressing themselves in Near, Far or Infinite space.

Practice 6: The Zen Garden

Group practice

Setting up the practice: The movement vocabulary is walking and stopping, standing, sitting and lying down. Using this practice, landscapes appear and dissolve through the alternation of simple shapes and their spatial relationships.

Benefit

This practice has the same stabilizing effect as working with space on the grid. The actors acquire a profound stability as their spatial and visual form develops in awareness. As a jazz musician is trained to listen to chords and notes, this practice trains the actor to listen to space and shape.

Practice 7: Corridors (conceived by Barbara Dilley)

Group practice

Setting up the practice: Establish parallel corridors, or paths, for each participant. The corridors can run from upstage to downstage, stage left to stage right.

The movement vocabulary is unrestricted in this practice, the performers work to establish visual, temporal and spatial dialogues.

Benefit

The use of the spatial restriction facilitates a highly complex compositional investigation.

Practice 8: Mandala (conceived by Barbara Dilley)

Group practice

Setting up the practice: Draw as large a circle as you can in the space. Then place a figure eight inside that is drawn large enough to touch the top and bottom of the enclosing circle. Then draw another figure eight of the same size but place it exactly perpendicular to the original figure eight. The two should meet and cross in the center of the design. At the apex of each of the four loops of the figure eights, draw a smaller circle. These smaller circles should also connect to the large original circle.

The pattern should be as big as possible to give the participants room to move freely. The participants walk, or establish other activities such as sitting, reading, knitting, or sleeping on the path of the mandala. The participants should not converse. The mandala should be performed for at least four hours and can be extended to any length that is desired.

Benefit

This practice brings the understanding that spatial patterns have a mysterious psychological and emotional effect on us.

Practice 9: Floor Pattern

Solo practice

Setting up the practice: Working with pen and paper.

Sitting at a table, create drawings on paper that can eventually be used as possible blocking or choreographic floor patterns. Use the drawing to create a series of patterns which are pleasing on their own. Bring the drawing into the studio and walk, dance or act a scene on the floor pattern.

Benefit

This practice encourages the use of space to go beyond its servitude to the choreography or the play. The act of drawing develops spatial skill and provides inspiration for imaginative staging. The drawings challenge and inform habitual or expedient staging.

Examples:

Use the drawing in a scale that is too large for the space.
Use the drawing to fill only one small area of the stage, leaving the rest empty.

Shape Practices

Practice 1: Solo Shape

Solo practice

Setting up the practice: The performer brings their attention to their body. It is important to make clear that no predesigned posture should be invented. Simply start with the sitting or standing posture you are in at the moment.

This practice involves studying the body through observation of symmetry, asymmetry, curved and bent shape, and relationships of one part of the body to the other. This observation is to last as long as the performer can hold their attention to find information from the position of their body. They should be told that they are simply collecting information at first. In order to do this the performer can lift and shift their head to take in all that is possible about the shapes they are observing in their body.

When the information begins to suggest a shift in shape, the performer should allow their body to make that shift according to the "voice" of the shape they are "hearing." As they settle into the "new" shape, a lengthy period of observation should again commence.

Benefit

A physical/visual awareness begins to build and with it the skill of performing even in stillness on stage. I have found that Shape awareness allows the performer to cross a threshold of intimacy while being watched, in which is instilled a calmness, assurance and elevating vulnerability.

Practice 2: Duet Shape 1-1

Duet practice

Setting up the practice: The performers should designate themselves as "One" and "Two." The performers then assume a shape; these shapes should not be approached as being acts of creativity in and of themselves.

Both performers hold their shape until a lengthy observation, first of Performer One and then of Performer Two, has ensued. Then Performer One should shift their shape and both performers commence observation again to bring their awareness to the new forms that have occurred in the duet.

After a lengthy period of observation, Performer Two shifts, followed by observation. In this way the practice continues, being careful to allow enough time for both parties to visually comprehend their own shape, the other performer's shape, and the conversation between the two.

In this practice, the quality of the shapes is of very little importance. The observation of the shapes carries the information and influence of this practice. If proper time is given to observation a mysterious transformation will occur: the shapes will begin to think for themselves.

In order to facilitate this phenomenon, the shapes should be of simple construction. The performers should be encouraged to move their heads, even though it may distort the shape, in order to facilitate maximum observation.

Benefit

This procedure allows for shape awareness to expand to include a larger conversation and to create a basis for partnership between performers. Once the performers are able to see well they can allow their timing to move faste,r and finally overlap without the restrictions of move-stop timing.

This work dramatically increases visual awareness of the body. When a performer acquires their own visual sense of themselves they are able to actively occupy stillness.

The activity they are performing is in the various languages of Shape. Another benefit of this practice is that it can make a performer much more visible onstage and gives the performer a great deal of material to work with in developing their character. This practice provides a rare opportunity for a performer, director, or choreographer to take time to observe form.

Practice 3: Temples

Duet practice

Setting up the practice: Focus on shapes to form structure out of two bodies. Both participants should maintain the same independence of solo shape practice and move-stop timing, used in Duet Shape 1-1 practice. The performers may physically connect the shapes but should avoid any situation where a partner is blocked from moving independently.

The difference between Temples and Duet Shape 1-1 is subtle but important. Duet Shape 1-1 is focused on observation and Temples is focused on using shape awareness to construct a performance in this material.

Benefit

This practice begins to lay the foundation for telling stories with shape. As the shapes progress the actors and dancers respond to a logic that is continually evolving. Different partners will find that they constitute a particular style and emotional world. Different partners make entirely different "stories." This lays the foundation for cooperation between individual styles.

Practice 4: Unison Shape

Group practice

Setting up the practice: Start with the group standing equally spread out over the room. The leader is the person who is farthest forward in the direction that the group is facing. Leadership changes when the group turns to face a different direction. If the group splits because of confusion allow the separate parts to work for a while and recombine if they want to. The movement given by the leaders should be slow enough for the group to have a chance to follow simultaneously.

The objective is to copy the movement as closely as possible. The actors should concentrate on details such as: the tension in the muscles, breath, the position of the fingers, the angle of the head, the timing, etc. As the practice evolves, any "mistakes" should be integrated into a cohesive whole that approximates the tone of the leader as closely a possible.

Benefit

This practice creates an immense sense of unity between performers if it is practiced over a period of a month or more. Through the act of observation and emulation, a bond is established that embraces the individual movement style and character of each performer. Unison Shape practice is foundational to ensemble work.

Practice 5: Moving Shapes

Solo practice

Setting up the practice: Create a shape with your body and press yourself to find out how it will move through space.

This is a very stiff and inconvenient approach to working. It does not feel good. It is frustrating. It makes you feel like you can't move and never did move well, but it is very educational. The shape begins to show you how it wants to move through space. In contemplating a shape, the arms may indicate a slide through space in a particular direction, or the tilt of the head may lead you, or the knee might bring you to the floor.

Benefit

This practice starts to relate shape to space and movement. In approaching the work in this way, the shape dialogue is put first and then ties back into the other components.

Practice 6: Fluid Shape Awareness

Solo practice

Setting up the practice: Imagine a highly mobile movie camera that is traveling rapidly around your body in every possible direction and angle. Begin moving, place your focus into the camera, and follow the shapes that flow out of your body. Move before you think.

Many shapes will escape before you become aware of them. However, the challenge will sharpen your ability to remain aware of your shapes even while in motion.

Benefit

This practice develops a very acute awareness of shape while in motion. It has a startling ability to make performers highly visible onstage while in motion.

Time Practices

Practice 1: Walking and Stopping, Time Awareness

Solo and group practice

Setting up the practice: The movement vocabulary is walking and stopping and as with the Walk and Stop for spatial practice, no other body movements should be used.

Staying with the simple unarticulated body, refrain from using the arms to make shapes or gestures; refrain from bending to the floor; refrain from using kinetics. This ensures that your concentration remains on time. The subject of this work is focusing on length of time standing, length of time walking, and composing with these elements. This work cannot be rushed or forced into manifesting itself. In some strange way, this work is most effective if it is approached with the sensual quality of "feeling" time. In order to work with time you must be able to stay in time rather than indicate it. Every muscle, fiber, and brain cell has to be precisely committed to the time you are in. In articulating time, you cannot allow your attention to wander into a relaxed state in which you are temporarily unaware of time. This does not mean that you cannot be casual, even lethargic, but if your attention is even a hair's breath off you are not translating the time into time awareness; you are not "doing time"—you are simply occupying it as would any non-performer.

This would be like pointing in a general direction and saying "put the couch somewhere over there" when designing the space in your apartment.

I have found that working with time has a more powerful emotional charge than any of the other SSTEMS. Perhaps this is because of the immense pressure that we put on time to civilize us and bring us under control. Or perhaps it is because time is connected to our central nervous system. We are hypersensitive to circumstances in which a new time has been introduced or invented.

Benefit

This practice builds awareness of options and depth of articulation. It is also very good as an ensemble-building technique. Working with time physically cultivates some of the most accurate uses of the body.

Practice 2: Repetition

Solo practice, which can, in some instances, be brought to group work

Setting up the practice: Set up a gesture, movement combination or text which you can repeat.

This practice sets up conditions in which you can focus on gradual changes in timing. As the repetition of a movement or text continues, notice that time can begin to shift, become shortened or stretched, fracture or slide together.

Benefit

This work allows the performer to experience time in a controlled study that reveals the subtlety and nuance that time is capable of producing. This work can affect speech patterns, line delivery, movement emphasis, and articulation of meaning both textually or choreographically.

Practice 3: Follow-Up on Repetition

Solo and group practice

Setting up of the practice: In this practice the vocabulary should include all six languages: Space, Shape, Time, Movement, Emotion, and Story. Repetition can be explored by using any or all of the SSTEMS, picking up and dropping any action at will.

This is an open improvisation with emphasis on options for repetition using any of the Six Viewpoints in combination or one at a time.

Benefit

The flow from repetition to open improvisation is a valuable learning tool. In the study of time it is very important to integrate repetition into a larger framework for greater facility and awareness of time. Repetition is a valuable tool in shaping logic and structure.

Practice 4: Unusual Time

Solo and group practice

Setting up the practice: As a group or alone, come up with descriptive words such as smashed, folded, stretched, dripping, etc. Use the time indicated in these words as generators of your actions.

This is a word game challenging our very limited time vocabulary. We have very few words for various speeds of motion. We have more words for how we like our steak cooked. Compare fast and slow to rare, medium rare, medium, done, well done. We all know that clouds have a certain time signature, cloud time. Air escaping from a carbonated drink when it is opened has a timing, ffffft time. Gusting winds follow a certain kind of timing that is like an attack and then a suspension. Pendulum action maintains a certain kind of timing which entropies as it progresses. Cats have a certain timing as do dogs, horses, trout, and refrigerator motors; however, we have not familiarized ourselves enough with them to bring them into our time vocabulary.

Benefit

This work should start a process of awareness of timing, time qualities and time invention.

This practice pushes time toward a new world. When sensitized to time, actors and dancers can begin to use it as part of their character, as a coordinator with other performers, and as an analytical tool for understanding a scene. This work radically improves physical movement acuity in performance. The effect of working in unusual time cultivates amazing physical accuracy and can establish a broad, expansive foundation for impulse work.

Practice 5: Developing Courage

Solo and group practice

Setting up the practice: Set up studies in which time is the center of the exploration. Do five gestures in five minutes.

Do 13 movements or gestures in one minute, one movement or gesture in the next minute, and use this cycle to build a scene.

Make a scene or a dance that is slightly slower than normal, but not in slow motion.

Give yourself permission to take a long time to think about what you want to do and then finally do it.

There is a common belief in theater and dance that you must keep your audience "entertained." This usually translates into an urge to fill every moment of the performance with activity and information. Actors, dancers, choreographers, and directors have a fear of stillness. Many people see stillness as emptiness. In working with time it is very important to get past these ideas and establish an authority with timing, stillness, or non-activity so that your range of expression is not constantly in high gear.

Benefit

This practice breaks down unconscious prejudices and fears about time. This may sound funny, but it really works to build confidence as a performer, director and choreographer.

Practice 6: Cartoon Coordination

Solo, duet, trio and group practice

Setting up the practice: Set up a movement or scene, then go about performing the movement or scene with every possible, and as many changes of rhythm you can imagine. It is helpful to think about the movement of cartoon characters. Cartoon movement is achieved by pixelation—a performer executing stop motion—but in this case, radical changes of time are inserted frame by frame.

Benefit

This practice allows coordination of different timings and breaks habitual use of time, or as I like to put it, neglect of time. Strangely enough, this work allows time to sink into the body as a natural expressive material.

Practice 7: Time Line

Solo and group practice

Setting up the practice: Set out a linear path on the floor. The performers decide how many steps long the path is (18 is a good number). When done in a group each performer has their own line. These lines can be parallel or otherwise. Walking only, begin to create rhythm patterns by counting the number of steps, then turning and counting the steps you take back. For instance, you might start with four steps, turn and take one step, turn and take four, and then turn and take one. In that way you can work out a huge variety of counts and patterns. As you work keep the rhythm of the walking and turning in the same beat.

This practice is actually a part of a process invented by choreographer Judy Padow. She made many variations on this form. During the time that I was in her company we must have covered thousands of miles in rehearsing this mesmerizing work.

Benefit

This practice provides accuracy with time measurement and patterning of motion.

Emotion Practices

Practice 1: Presence Work

Solo practice

Setting up the practice: Set a chair in the middle of the space. Sit a person in the chair. Watch them. The performer should attempt to maintain all normal habits such as blinking, breathing, thinking, emotional reactions, twitches, attention shifts, or swallowing.

The minimum time needed to sit in this observed study is five minutes. The longer the performer can be there the more profound the experience. I recommend sitting for 20 minutes to get the full experience.

The performer should be instructed to neither avoid looking at the audience nor look at them too much in self-defense. They should allow themselves to be seen.

They are permitted to move around in the space, but I have found that the chair and the activity of sitting help establish a vulnerability and normalcy to the event that standing and walking can complicate.

Benefit

The performer starts to be able to surrender to the audience and to appreciate being watched. Their being becomes larger and stronger. They can make friends with the audience, which is profound. It is quite surprising how many performers do not really like the audience and feel that they must protect themselves from the people they perform for.

There is also a profound benefit for the rest of the class. In the act of impersonating the audience, the rest of the performers are allowed to see how profoundly interesting and moving the performer is in and of themselves.

As the time passes, and if everything goes well, the "audience" starts to see through the performer straight to something that looks like the soul. This is an earthshaking experience for many performers and directors.

The power of looking into someone is very evident as it stands before you in the studio or theater. The most revolutionary thing is that this power is arrived at without real determined effort by the performer. It's the performer's acceptance and willingness to open up to the underlying reality of being onstage, and being looked at, and unable to hide, that creates what we call presence.

Practice 2: Emotional Walk and Stop

Solo and group practice

Setting up the practice: The setup of movement restrictions are the same as the original Walk and Stop. While using the spatial dialogue of the original practice, the performer should take on a secondary focus by collecting emotional information. This is done by asking the question "how does standing in this place feel emotionally?"

The performer should ask:

How does it feel to stand this close to the wall? How does this diagonal feel?

How does it feel to be this close to the audience? How does it feel to be all the way up stage?

How does it feel to have my back to the audience?

How does it feel to be this close or distant to the other performers? How does it feel to stand at this angle to the other performer or performers?

How does it feel to walk in this pattern in relationship to the other performers?

How does being stationary feel while everyone else is moving? How does my spatial placement and patterning build a character in relationship to the other characters?

What should my next move be in relationship to what I am feeling with the group?

Most performers naturally gravitate to the center of the stage and stay there. There is a good reason for this. They instinctually know that they are standing in the most important and commanding spot that the stage has to offer. They know that if they stand there they will be able to have emotional command of the audience's attention, because they are making the statement, just as a child would, "I am the most important thing in your life."

Because of the demands of this work, it should be approached with patience and low expectations in the beginning so that the coordination of these voices can be integrated.

Benefit

With this practice the performer, director and choreographer obtain a broader view of the emotional implications of space. They expand their space vocabulary, and build up confidence that different positions onstage have emotional messages that can support the text and movements, or actually evoke the emotion needed at that moment. In this practice the group can slowly build an emotional atmosphere that is not driven by an outside motivation. The work helps to educate the performers that the emotional context of their being onstage is a real entity that can begin to suggest its own emotional logic. This work is also good for building ensemble skills, and lays a foundation for giving and taking stage focus among performers. The work can generate the understanding in directors and choreographers that emotional nuance can build with great precision when the language of emotion is researched outside the project that the artist is focusing on.

Practice 3: Open Emotional Improvisation

Group practice

Setting up the practice: In an open movement vocabulary, using all the SSTEMS, the performers should be told to explore doing anything they like that occurs to them on an emotional level. Before they begin work they should be told to stay with what they are feeling for as long and only as long as they want. A performer should not take responsibility for any other person's emotional needs. They need to have the freedom to slide from one emotion to another without any logical connection or commitment to anything they are doing.

This work requires a special warm up which will take the performers past judgment.

I recommend the lower brain, child developmental patterns in the work of Bonnie Bainbridge Cohen, or any type of work that takes the performer past rational judgment as they move their bodies. The performers need to suspend their normal adult reserve and be willing to become childlike and make fools of themselves.

Benefit

This practice allows the emotional vocabulary to expand into unlabeled emotional situations. Because it is not focused on achieving anything, even control, the performers can gain confidence in the "performance" of emotions. As the performers work in this practice, they build an understanding of emotional interaction which is based on a primal attention span rather than out of social or artfully constructed obligation. I have found that this practice builds emotional timing, and quickens emotional reflexes.

Movement Practices

Practice 1: Kinetic Feedback/Doing What the Body Wants

Solo practice

Setting up the practice: Standing in a studio, bring your concentration to the level of sensation in your body. Allow your body to move from sensation and to move to create sensation. Allow the sensory dialogue to flow in a stream of consciousness. Observe how a kinetic logic begins to evolve and set up. Attune yourself to gravity, pendulum action, balance, muscle tension, touch, etc. A more complete source for this work can be found in chapter 5, Movement.

This practice derives movement from sensation and is the basic Viewpoints practice for isolating and dialoguing with movement.

Benefit

This work will not create very beautiful movement. The practice should not be used to derive movement, invention, or creation. It is designed to strengthen the link between body, feeling, and action. When this practice is assimilated, movements will become more fully invested. This investment can then be applied to any form. Actors will find that this practice brings the entire subject of movement in performance to life.

Practice 2: Lower Brain Movement

Solo practice

Setting up the practice: The first stages of this work should begin with lying on the floor on your back. In this position, allow your mind to come to a blank and give yourself the instruction that you would like your body to move from impulse rather than from a thought-out command. Usually this work comes out as very sharp movements that course through the body causing it to shudder, jump or jerk for a few seconds. Very quickly the mind catches up and begins to reflect on the movement. At that point the body and mind should be placed back to neutral and the process started again.

The work engages the automatic movement center located in the lower brain. I put this work together from classes I took with the teacher, artist, and dancer Beth Goren in her classes on Body-Mind Centering. This part of the brain is devoted to automatic movements such as breathing, heart rate, pulling your hand away from fire, and jumping out of the path of a speeding object. This is the purest form of the body creating its own movement, free of images, free of learned information, and free of planned designs.

Benefit

I have found that repeated practice in this form causes a wonderful sense of well-being and a startling connection between the mind and body. This practice causes the body to respond to thought processes with much greater accuracy and speed. Our movement is generally habituated to visual and spatial coordination. We are usually not allowed to move without thinking. This causes the movement response to partially fall asleep, relying on other parts of the brain as it senses and directs movement.

Practice 3: Kinetic Duets

Duet practice

Setting up the practice: Use your partner's movement as a stimulus for your own movement.

The work deals with the Duet form that is very like the Duet Shape practice. This requires a level of moving before thinking, stimulated by the lower brain movement practice. In this case, the performer should try to move just a few seconds ahead of the mind, allowing it to follow slightly behind as an observer. There is a tendency for this practice to escalate in speed and size. The performers should be reminded that they can focus on subtle kinetic sensations and movements and use variations of speed and size.

Benefit

This work is excellent for training the eye to kinetic feedback and dialogue. It also is very good for movement invention.

The late musician, teacher, and conceptualist Robert Dunn had practices that were similar to this. He would first have the dancers generate raw material from suggestions such as sink, roll, and pause. After the dancers worked for some time he would then begin to introduce an editing process by having the performers select movements that they found particularly interesting. The selected material would then become the starting point for another improvisation. This selection process would continue until the material was distilled into very focused subject matter.

Practice 4: Doing the Unnecessary

Solo practice

Setting up the practice: Use too much or too little energy and or muscle tension for a given movement. Work toward illogical patterns of movement rather than logical flow. For instance: fall in seven steps, change direction, speed and kinesthetic language at each step. Do not work with the organic. Counter every logical move.

This practice came from a dance I worked on from 1997 to 1999. It is now a major part of my teaching of the Six Viewpoints.

Benefit

This looking beyond the logical, the organic, the natural causes a big expansion in movement vocabulary and can also be very humorous. Performers derive the ability to play with anything, make anything into art by recognizing its value. This practice wakes up the brain like nothing I have ever encountered. At this point in my teaching, this is my most treasured practice.

Practice 5: Body Parts

Solo practice

Setting up the practice: Select two body parts and work them in pairs as movement sources: hand and head, foot and mouth, spine and knee, knee and pelvis, elbow and neck, etc. The potential pairings of body parts, as you can imagine, numbers in the hundreds.

Benefit

This work brings the body into a world that has been lost to us as we strive to train movement facility through various techniques such as ballet, modern and even the pre-movement trainings of postmodern dance. Those techniques can inhibit new movement inventions and sensation. The Body Parts practice can simultaneously humble and amaze performers with the possibilities of the movement of our bodies. This practice leaves the actor or dancer with the question, what else could happen?—a satisfying affirmation that movement is infinite.

Practice 6: The Hands Come Together and the Feet Run Parallel

Group practice

Setting up the practice: The title is the instruction for this practice.

These instructions form a mysterious set of physical activities. This is like working on a play with only half a plot. The movement that arises from trying to resolve these directions results in an outpouring of action as the performer works on the unsolvable logic.

Benefit

The most exciting attribute of this practice is that it is a movement puzzle that cannot be solved, and the longer you play with it, the more combinations arise to befuddle you. Because of this, it shakes the performer away from the restrictive idea of doing the practice correctly.

Story Practices

Practice 1: Group Story Improvisation

Group practice

Setting up the practice: Begin with everyone following a solo storyline at the same time. Use story as a kind of fourth-dimensional surfboard; allow the story to include any material, to change at any time, go in any direction, switch radically, end or evolve. Practice letting the story go but keeping up with where it is going. Instead of controlling the story, allow it to wander.

As the multiple solo stories fill the room avoid getting into any other story but your own. As you come across the other performers they must be woven into your own story. If you find yourself confused or at a loss, then bridge the moment by including the pause or your confusion in the stream of the story. Do not create a narration—the stories should come into your mind and body on their own. Your practice is one of letting go and following.

A sample storyline that came out of this practice: "The washcloth came to rest at the bottom of the sea, all time left him and he became a plastic ball as a large fish swept over him."

Benefit

This practice brings two strengths to the story language:
  (1) develops story concentration, individuation and independence
  (2) increases tolerance and the ability to function in a multi-dimensional story environment

In reality, we only have our story and follow it without break in a sea of other stories, stories which we only partly understand at best, but with which we must interact. An independent performer enriches everyone's experience by adding the dimension of their own understanding of what they are performing.

Practice 2: Multidimensional Stories

Solo and group practice

Setting up the practice: Construct a story using the exploratory process explained below. Work on each step of this process separately and then combine the pieces into one composition.

Construct a logic progression using only spatial patterns.

Compose a logic structure that uses unusual time and a known script. Layer the script with three different or opposing motivations.

Compose the story backwards.

This practice is best done over a series of days to give the logic process time to be in dialogue. It is important to remember that you do not have to know what the story is until you are close to finishing the work. In this practice you find the logic and meaning through juxtaposition. The important thing is to follow your understanding of the logic as closely as you can.

Benefit

This practices provides experience in multi-dimensional logic and by understanding that there is more than one way to tell a story.

Practice 3: Image Work

Solo practice

Setting up the practice: Present the performers with the following list: white wall, coat hanger, wastepaper basket, man's suit, or refrigerator. Choose one of the images and improvise with it physically for 10 to 20 minutes. Perform the work for the group.

Benefit

This practice is a path to finding new stories. I have found that subjects holding very little information or potential reveal that we have a greater knowledge of stories than we suspect. I have used this practice for many years as a vital component of my classroom training.

This practice will bring out information that you did not know you held in your Story brain. We actually know a great deal more about refrigerators than we suspect. The point of this experience is to find stories in places where we had no idea there were stories. This practice allows the student to understand that delightful and moving stories are hiding everywhere.

Practice 4: Finding a Story

Solo and group practice

Setting up the practice: Choose a topic such as the ones listed below. Find a place to start in any of these stories and tell it. You might choose to tell the story, using only small details, from the point of view of the sidewalk, or from the middle progressing simultaneously to the beginning and to the end.

the story of a nation

the story of man

the story of woman

the story of snow

the story of my pair of black shoes

the story of our steaks

the story of our dinner together

The postmodern idea of story is that it comes about through presentation of logic that can emerge from many different perspectives. The logic does not have to depend on "beginning, middle, and end" for strength and validity.

Benefit

Whether telling new stories or old ones, the practice of seeing subtlety and fluidity of story structures is beneficial for performers, directors, choreographers, and dancers. This practice also instills confidence in storytelling and logic construction through experimentation.

Improvisations

The last practices of The Viewpoints address the wonderful resource that improvisation brings to performance.

Improvisation is a large part our lives. Every day we grapple with a flood of unpredictable information and try to organize it into some comprehensible logic. The challenge of improvisation is to cross-pollinate events in the moment with all that we have already mastered. In my mind, this process produces the most sophisticated art. In the world of art, improvisation challenges the known by extending sound, form, physicality, the visual, and meaning to discover what exists at the edges of our comprehension.

For improvisation to be of value the seminal challenge is the issue of control. Why so, one asks, since it seems to be based on anything goes? The issue of control arises because improvisation still has to contain comprehensible logic, both for the audience, and for the performers themselves. There needs to be logic even in improvisation because what we can't read, we can't use or respond to.

Practice 1: Doing the Unnecessary

Solo and group practice

Setting up the practice: Enter the studio practice room. Acknowledge that in life we carefully and slowly learn to be effective and efficient in accomplishing daily tasks, such as walking, sitting, leaving a room, dressing, drinking from a cup. Then acknowledge that you are about to practice forgetting how to do these daily tasks. If you should reach out to turn the doorknob as you prepare to leave the room, turn yourself instead, try singing a song to get the door open, try to get someone on the other side to open the door. If you want to sit in a chair to read a book, stand near it and read your book upside down and backwards while pushing the chair out of reach each time you attempt to sit in it. When this work is done within a group, performers are permitted to be obstructive, non-cooperative, or just minimally cooperative. I allow this practice to extend for at least 40 minutes to over an hour. Our ability to find and perform the unnecessary is practically inexhaustible once you catch onto the idea.

Benefit

The discovery of the Unnecessary was my final epiphany, bringing about the Laboratory of the Original Anarchist. Many aspects of making art are very hard, sometimes even grim: searching out a subject, choosing the right logic, caring for the details, the physical labor of production. And while these are labors of love they are labors nonetheless. Doing the Unnecessary is a totally joyous holiday for the artist. Yet, while "on vacation," the mind is trained to be incredibly alert—because if we are not vigilant, we will automatically return to the necessary. We have labored hard in our lives to be efficient, coordinated, and practical. Throwing this ingrained habit overboard lands us in a world of invention that is infinite and secured in "right action" because it is allowed to function simply on a level of physicality

We glide to the end. I hope you have enjoyed being in the studio with some of these practices. I know that I never tire of them. This last is one dearest to my heart. It came as the product of a lifetime devoted to these practices.

Most performers treat the stage as though it is a pool table. Each has the project of playing the ball (line or action) into the pocket with skill and efficiency. The problem with this skilled performance is that as the show proceeds there are fewer and fewer balls on the table, fewer things to play, and energy is draining off the table/stage because of the pocketing of the balls. The poor performer has to increase the energy of their performance in order to compensate for this problem. Pool on an Egg-Shaped Table is meant to compensate for this traditional game-of-pool process.

Practice 2: Pool on an Egg-Shaped Table

Group practice

Setting up the practice: Each performer adopts a singular, non-inclusive focus, metaphorically turning their back on the other performers. Participants may not use any material other than their own, and may not relate to others in time, gesture or in any other manner. The project is to generate all your own material. The practice is united by the thinnest connection: occasionally the participants are required to glance over their shoulders to check out what is going on in the room. If, coincidentally, cooperation occurs, it is permissible to pursue it, but only until your own logic finds a way out.

The table is the shape of an eggshell cut in half. Can you visualize this? Cup your hand holding the palm up to the ceiling. This is the position and approximate shape of the egg-shaped table. Because of its cupped egg shape, it is impossible to predict the outcome of your or anyone's actions.

Benefit

This type of performance never runs out of material. The practice stretches the ability to explain, rationalize and discover art. Playing Pool on an Egg-Shaped Table makes you very independent. I believe that many principles found in Chaos Theory are present in the practice.

Acknowledgments

In the decades it took to produce this book, there have been seven versions completed and set aside as not good enough. Although not one word has been written by someone other than me, nine people have been important to this process as editors or advisers. Lisa Nelson of Contact Quarterly assisted me in establishing a writing voice and style. William Daddario, while still a student at the Experimental Theatre Wing, collaborated with me on establishing a linear organization the material. Branislav Jokovic coached me on how to remove words. Ben Yalom coached me on the value of stories and metaphors, a writing technique I was very reluctant to employ but finally learned to use on my own terms. The late Nicole Potter helped to tame my writhing repetitive text. Johanna Rosenbaum and Michael Levine pressed me to clarify the titles of the sections of the Bridge. Joe Gill spent hours reading and cleaning a version with me. Catherine Courtenaye put the finishing touches on the text to achieve a lovely and delicate clarity.

My gratitude to all the teachers, choreographers, directors, actors and dancers who have found merit in using my work over the years. A special thanks to Wendell Beavers for his years of promoting and teaching the Viewpoints.

My gratitude to the people who have supported me in the process of being an artist and of writing: the late Gennie and Robert DeWeese, Tina DeWeese Kate Bradley, Deborah White, Donna Lingle, Paul Langland, Jan Wenk, Terry O'Reilly, Lee Breuer, Ruth Maleczech, Carol McDowell, Ismael Ivo, Carl Regensburger, Herta Straka, Nanc Allen, Rosemary Quinn, Lisa Sokolov, Terry Knickerbocker, Jonathan Hart, Louise Scheeder, Mary Campbell Smith, Kevin Kuhlke, Arthur Bartow, Colin Cochran, Barney O'Hanlon, Timothy Scott, Nicolas Norena, Hanna Gross and Janice Orlandi.

My gratitude to a secret coven for contributing sustenance through mutual interest and engagement with whatever we were thinking about: Nina Martin, Cynthia Hedstrom, Erica Fae and Sophia Treanor. I am sure that when I die your names will be found etched in my bones.

Finally, there are no words of gratitude that could possibly express a very special thank you to Sally Sommers for recommending me to Ron Argelander when he was looking to hire, in 1978, the first teacher for the Experimental Theatre Wing at Undergraduate Drama Tisch School of the Arts at New York University, in doing so she managed to create a wonderful home for the Viewpoints.

MARY OVERLIE

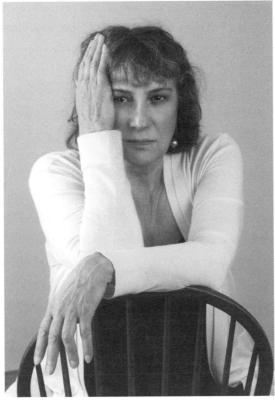

NORTHERN SUMMIT STUDIO

Mary Overlie

What can you say about a person who at an early age discovered that she would be content to spend 90 percent of her life in a closet thinking, yet who thought nothing of hopping a freight train to Berkeley, California at the age of 17 with only $50 dollars in her pocket, to pursue dancing?

Mary Overlie is an observer/participant, a deconstructing postmodern theatre practitioner, an original anarchist. She is a woman who is not afraid of obscurity, or worried that being unknown might obscure her ideas. She prefers to remain out of the limelight in order to create. She has a deep trust and confidence in a piercing mind. At a young age she displayed an intense physical and intellectual confidence. The Theory and Practice of The Six Viewpoints were borne out that confidence with a quiet yet infectious impact.

"Observe the ingredients, the materials of performance, contemplate the particles. Once you find them, train yourself to listen, allow them to become your teachers, embrace them as profound partners. Allow them to create."

Any theater artist standing in Overlie's classroom is immediately drawn to her clarity: able to absorb, comprehend and take her teachings to heart. Throughout her many years of teaching, she has managed to articulate a very basic and functional view and practice of postmodern art. Her views on performance are clear and resilient as the views and grass on the high prairie.

Overlie was born January 15, 1946 in Terry, Montana; conceived MOVEMENT RESEARCH, a cooperative dance organization of international renown; founded DANSPACE PROJECT with BARBARA DILLEY, a dance presenting organization in New York City; first teacher hired to establish the EXPERIMENTAL THEATRE WING AT TISCH SCHOOL OF THE ARTS AT NEW YORK UNIVERSITY; a choreographer and performer with an international reputation in the field of experimental dance, for many years teaching and performing as a part of the INTERNATIONAL TANZ WOCHEN working with ISMAEL IVO AND KARL REGENSBURGER in Vienna. Recently retired after 39 years teaching in the Undergraduate Drama Department at NYU she now resides in Bozeman, Montana.

THE SIX VIEWPOINTS is her child and it has done a unique thing in the world of theater and performance philosophy; it has come with a quiet and infectious ability to represent itself without her. She joins those who have worked to elevate theater. Her leveling of the creative hierarchy by focusing on the materials has conceptually and practically infected the performance worlds of both theater and dance.